MOM, SAVE MY BRAIN

THE HIDDEN AIRWAY CRISIS CAUSING BRAIN DYSFUNCTION IN HUNDREDS OF MILLIONS OF CHILDREN WORLDWIDE

CANDY SPARKS

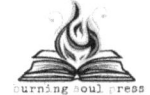
burning soul press

Paperback: 978-1-964924-12-0
Hardcover: 978-1-964924-13-7
eBook: 978-1-964924-14-4

CONTENTS

TESTIMONIALS

"A mother's determination to navigate complex medical systems and secure life-changing treatment for her daughter… essential reading for parents and healthcare workers alike."

SURESH KOTAGAL M.D., PEDIATRIC NEUROLOGIST AND SLEEP SPECIALIST

"All prospective parents must read this book to avoid the airway epidemic we face! Thank you, Candy Sparks, for bringing this valued information to the public awareness!"

JOY L. MOELLER, BS, RDH, AOMT-C, CERTIFIED OROFACIAL MYOFUNCTIONAL THERAPIST

"Early detection of airway obstruction in newborns is absolutely critical. Without immediate intervention, these children face risks of brain injury, neuromuscular disorders, and even death. We urgently need a universal screening protocol that ensures every newborn's airway is properly assessed. Candy Sparks' *Mom Save My Brain* is a crucial wake-up call to both medical professionals and parents. Her work illuminates a path forward, showing how getting this right in those first crucial moments can make the difference between a child thriving or suffering lifelong complications."

DR. LARRY WOLFORD, DMD, LEADING
ORAL AND MAXILLOFACIAL SURGEON

"Candy Sparks' new book, *Mom Save My Brain*, sheds a bright, new light on a critical public health problem. Recognized over 100 years ago, but essentially ignored until recently, this problem puts millions of children at risk for permanent brain damage. Learn about simple signs easily recognized by parents (but often ignored by well-meaning but uninformed health care providers) which can identify children at risk. The SAT Prep you fund for your high school student isn't likely to make up for the brain damage that might have been prevented when your child was 3 years old. This book is a must-read for all parents."

WILLIAM M. HANG, DDS, MSD,
ORTHO2HEALTH LINKEDIN

"All parents should read this book from cover to cover and then read it again!"

"Mom, Save My Brain is a compelling and essential read. As a sleep epidemiologist, I know that sleep is a cornerstone of healthy development in children, and compromised airways often undermine this crucial foundation. Candy Sparks' book not only highlights the challenges faced by families grappling with these under-recognized disorders but also underscores the urgent need for early screening, prevention, and treatment.

With invaluable resources for caregivers, healthcare providers, researchers, and public health professionals, *Mom, Save My Brain* serves as a call to action to address this significant public health burden. Candy Sparks' work is a testament to the critical need for awareness and advocacy in reducing the impact of airway disorders on children and their families.

I wholeheartedly recommend this book to anyone invested in improving child health and well-being. It is both inspiring and informative, offering hope and practical guidance to those navigating similar journeys."

"I see so much potential, not just for the good our work can do around the world, but for the good around the world that will be done by the children who benefit from this health crisis intervention."

SHAWN SÉKOU BONNEY, DIRECTOR,
CAFF EARLY CHILDHOOD
DEVELOPMENT

PREFACE

By Suresh Kotagal, M.D.
Emeritus Professor, Department of Neurology
Consultant in Pediatrics, Neurology and Sleep Medicine
(retired)
Mayo Clinic, Rochester, Minnesota

Narrowing or blockages in the upper airway that lead to its collapse during sleep, consequent obstructive sleep apnea (OSA), and consequent drops in blood oxygen levels are not readily detected early on in childhood. There are many reasons for this, including the fact that narrowing is not easily visible to parents and health care providers alike. Further, snoring, which frequently accompanies OSA in adults, is not always present in children. Primary care doctors are not always aware of this group of disorders from the standpoint of how to examine the patient, what tests to run, and what treatments to offer. There are many explanations behind this, but one that is easily identified is the lack of exposure to these disorders during medical school education or residency training.

Childhood OSA can result from abnormal shape and small size of the upper airway, enlarged tonsils (at the back of the throat), enlarged adenoids (at the back of the nasal passages), obesity, and neuromuscular disorders (like muscular dystrophy). Roughly two percent of children have OSA. Due to a lack of awareness amongst parents and healthcare providers alike, childhood OSA can go unrecognized and untreated for months to years. An important consequence of OSA is recurrent drops in blood oxygen levels or increases in carbon dioxide levels during sleep. This nightly abnormality in the quality of blood gases occurs at a young age while the brain is actively developing its network of synaptic connections that are crucial for learning new concepts and the appropriate control of behavior. Untreated OSA in preschool-age children can lead to behavioral problems such as poor attention span and hyperactivity. As a consequence, a child may end up mistakenly diagnosed as having attention deficit hyperactivity disorder (ADHD) and receive treatment with stimulants like methylphenidate. The irony is that all the while the underlying culprit of OSA remains undetected and untreated. This is a tragedy because definitive treatments do exist; the most common is a surgery called tonsillectomy or adenotonsillectomy, which opens the upper airway space to counterbalance the tendency for the airway to collapse during sleep. Dental devices that prevent the tongue from falling back and blocking the airway or those aimed at gradually opening up the nasal passages (maxillary distraction devices) are also available. Unless a child is lucky enough to see an upper airway specialist such as a pediatric otolaryngologist, pediatric orthodontist, or pediatric sleep specialist, the problem of upper airway collapse during sleep from OSA does not receive timely attention.

This is the unfortunate story of childhood OSA, especially when it is outwardly subtle and not recognized in time.

Though treatments are available, neither parents nor most health care providers may be aware of what steps they need to take to help a child. The author, Candy, paints a vivid picture of the numerous hoops that she and her husband had to jump through to get definitive and disease-modifying treatment for their daughter, Savvy. Candy's courage and dogged determination to get the appropriate help for her child is nothing but remarkable. In her search for what would be the best management approach for her child, in this book, we learn about Candy's experiences as she reaches out to many world-class specialists from dental sleep medicine, pediatrics, pediatric sleep medicine, otolaryngology, and myofunctional medicine who are able to finally help her daughter. I am also impressed by the discussion on newborn screening. If pediatricians can universally develop and follow an algorithmic approach to assessment and management of sleep-related obstructive airway problems during infancy before adverse consequences take hold, we might be able to save children and their parents a lot of unnecessary suffering later on in life.

Savvy's OSA was complicated by the presence of underlying Ehlers-Danlos syndrome (EDS), a connective tissue disorder that leads to laxity in joints and low muscle tone. Now that it has been discovered to be related to mutations in the COL5A2 gene, hopefully, one day, there will be a specific treatment available for EDS as well. In the words of Orison Swett Marden, an inspirational author who grew up during the nineteenth century in a poor farming community in New Hampshire, *"There is no medicine like hope, no incentive so great, and no tonic so powerful as the expectation of something tomorrow."*

INTRODUCTION

One day in 2011, when my daughter Savvy was just nine years of age, she came to me with a look of utter sadness and said, "Mom, I feel like my body is rotting, and I can no longer remember much of my childhood." She started to cry and said, "I don't know what's happening. I used to be smart and love to run. Now my mind is foggy, and I can't keep up with my friends anymore."

Can you imagine your child teetering on the edge of depression as they tell you that they feel like their body is rotting and that they're losing their memory?

Suddenly, nothing was more important to me than getting her the help she needed so she no longer felt an ounce of that. Unfortunately for us, Savvy already had significant hypoxic and systemic damage before we realized what was happening to her.

Savvy's early years gave no indication of the medical maelstrom that lay ahead. But subtle signs—restless sleeping, teeth grinding, snoring, and mouth breathing—gradually escalated into a debilitating condition that medical professionals failed to diagnose for over a decade. Savvy was journeying through a little-known and under-recognized realm of airway health disorders before my eyes, and I had no clue that this world existed. It's a world where breathing, sleep, and oral health are intricately connected to overall well-being, and yet the majority of parents in the U.S. aren't informed about this.

An alarming 400 million children across the globe, including millions in the United States, Europe, and Asia, grapple with compromised airways that severely impair their sleep, growth, behavior, and overall quality of life.[1] The impact of these disorders in childhood and adolescence carries into adulthood, so it's not just about raising healthy children, but, essentially, raising healthy adults as well.

Despite the staggering statistics showing that 11 million children under ten years old in the US, 250 million in Asia, 1.9 million in the UK, and 700,000 in Australia, among others, live with this burden, airway disorders remain enigmatic and often overlooked.[2] Their symptoms, seemingly negligible at first—subtle signs easy to dismiss or attribute to other factors —belies a condition that can drastically affect a child's sleep, growth, academic performance, physical health, behavior, and quality of life if left untreated.

My daughter Savvy's story is a poignant illustration of the insidious progression when an airway disorder is not caught early.

I thought I had done everything right. My pregnancy was very easy and went full-term. I never drank alcohol, smoked, or took any type of prescription or recreational drug. Our beautiful girl was a bouncing eight pounds, nine ounces at birth.

I breastfed Savvy until she was thirty-two months old. We traveled so often to see family from coast to coast that it was always easier for me to feed her on demand and not have to carry bottles. She hit all of her milestones early and was incredibly articulate and bright. We couldn't imagine that anything could be wrong.

However, at eighteen months, my leading cosmetic dentist, Dr. Brian McKay, saw her for just a minute in his office and said, "She is going to need some work as she gets older. There is a Dr. Bill Hang in California. You should take her there around six years of age."

I looked at my cute, brilliant daughter and thought, *What can he possibly mean? Oh well, I don't have to worry about it until she is six.* I know now that the highly trained eye of my cosmetic dentist saw a child who breathed through her mouth, had an accentuated cupid upper lip, a rolled lower lip, high dental arches, small jaws, and a facial structure common to those with compromised airways.

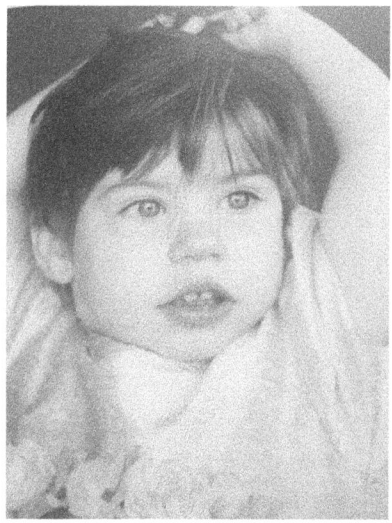

Her pediatricians did not see it. Her pediatric dentist did not see it, or if she had, she did not mention it. Even the emergency room doctors at Seattle Children's did not know what they were seeing. But the trained eye could readily see it and know that it would lead to a hypoxic brain injury—at the very least.

About a month after I stopped breastfeeding her, Savvy suddenly came down with pneumonia/RSV. (The doctors at Seattle Children's weren't quite sure which one it was.) Prior to this hospitalization, she had never been sick.

My next clue that something was off didn't come until Savvy was six when she collapsed while running a race. We immediately took her to a pediatric cardiologist and pediatric pulmonologist. Her heart and lungs checked out fine. At the time, we lived in Scottsdale. Our pediatrician suggested that maybe it was a light case of desert fever. Thankfully, she recovered quickly.

As Savvy's baby teeth fell out and her secondary teeth came in, they created an almost cartoonish grin known as a severe class II malocclusion. She could not close her mouth, and her mouth breathing became more evident.

What many parents are not aware of is that persistent mouth breathing results in about eighteen percent less oxygen reaching the brain.[3] Mouth breathing is one of the signs of an airway health disorder and severely interferes with quality of sleep, which, in turn, can also lower your child's IQ by as many as ten points compared to their IQ with proper sleep.[4] I had no idea at the time!

Having recently moved again as Savvy started third grade in Austin, Texas, her new classmates began to laugh at her cartoonish grin. We took her to see the highest rated local orthodontist. While there, we mentioned hearing about Dr. Hang in California and wondered if that was the next course of action. We were told that the orthodontist would be happy to discuss Savvy's case with Dr. Hang, but nothing would change. Savvy would need double jaw surgery, also known as orthognathic surgery (MMA), but could not have that done until she was fully grown, which is usually at the age of seventeen.

In the meantime, the orthodontist said he could give her a *nice smile*. A rapid expander was applied to her upper palate, and retractive orthodontic braces were placed on her teeth. Over the next several months, there were frequent appointments for adjustments.

What I know now is that even the loss of as little as two or three millimeters of space in the mouth caused by pushing the teeth back with retractive orthodontics can force the tongue farther back into the throat and block the airway. This is detrimental to those already showing signs of an airway disorder. That one move to "help" Savvy severely backfired.

About a year later, the braces were removed, and Savvy had a nice smile. But soon after, I attended her end-of-the-year fitness day celebration at school and witnessed, as she tried to jump rope for a minute, her collapse onto the floor. Looking almost like a fish out of water, she lay there gasping for air. She was humiliated and embarrassed. Later, she tried a relay race. She collapsed again.

We went immediately to her new pediatrician in Austin. He diagnosed exercise-induced asthma and prescribed inhalers. He told us to take Savvy to the track and do a run-walk routine several times per week. She was also found to be allergic to cedar trees.

However, during the exam, no one looked in her mouth and noticed the scalloped tongue, the worn teeth caused by grinding (also known as bruxism), or checked her partially blocked airway, even though she was mouth breathing.

That summer, I took her to Sweden to see friends and family. As we rushed through the airport, she could not keep up. She had to go slowly. We had no idea what was really taking place inside her.

It got worse. Wanting to play on the volleyball team with her friends, she began spraining her ankles frequently. We noticed then that her knees were developing abnormally, turning more inward. Her pediatrician recommended crutches like a bandaid, not looking into the actual problem of why this kept happening.

Savvy was on a downhill spiral. She could no longer remember to turn in her completed assignments and often zoned out in class. That's when we took her to Texas Children's in Houston to see the world-renowned pediatric pulmonologists seeking the definitive answers as to why Savvy couldn't seem to get enough air. Following an extensive examination, they said she was a *mystery*, prescribed even stronger inhalers, and recommended she reduce the stress of being at a very demanding prep school. No questions about sleep, collapsing, sprained ankles, knee issues, or mouth breathing were asked. They said she was likely stressed out and exhausted by her heavy school schedule.

In retrospect, someone with the trained eye would have noticed right away that she suffered from obstructive sleep apnea (OSA) and was beginning to show signs of ligamentous laxity and Hypermobile Ehlers-Danlos syndrome. When your brain and body are not getting enough oxygen because you breathe through your mouth, wake frequently, and cannot get the restorative sleep you need, your muscles do not develop properly to support your joints. Savvy's were beginning to dislocate. I now understand that compromised airways are often linked to muscle laxity, but the doctors we took her to at the time did not make that connection.

The following year, Savvy's best friend at school died from leukemia. He was the only one who told her that he recognized that she, too, was sick. She was not faking it, even though her friends and teachers were beginning to doubt her because she did not have a diagnosis or obvious physical signs. They could not see the blocked airway deep inside her mouth. They did not understand that with every passing day, it was more difficult to breathe. Worse, she could no longer keep pace walking across campus with her friends. She came late to classes because it took longer to climb the stairs. She was given her own key card to enter after everyone else had already made it to class.

Savvy was beginning to feel more ostracized and isolated. Depression was growing inside of her. She told me that she felt as though her body was rotting and she didn't know why she wasn't smart anymore. It was terrifying for her when she realized that she could no longer remember much of her childhood. At twelve years of age, she struggled to go on and wrote a suicide letter.

We consulted a friend who is a psychologist in Seattle, and our family flew up to meet with her. We also stopped to see Dr. Brian McKay, who has that extraordinarily well-trained eye. He examined Savvy by tipping her back in the dental chair and, while looking into her mouth, he said, "Oh my gosh! I don't know how she breathes! Her airway is fifty to eighty percent blocked. You must see Dr. Hang right away." We finally did. Dr. Hang prepared her for orthognathic surgery over the next six months.

She was only thirteen years of age. It was not possible to wait for surgery at seventeen. She would have been placed on CPAP for four years. I didn't feel we could steal another four years from her. During her meetings with the world-renowned maxillofacial surgeon Dr. Larry Wolford, she grew to trust him and desperately wanted to be able to breathe fully again.

On December 15, 2015, Savvy was one of the youngest people ever to have orthognathic surgery. On January 5, 2016, three weeks later, she was sitting on the curb outside of her new performing arts school, breathing fully and eagerly waiting to go in and start her life again. Things went well as she was able to go back half-time and rest as her body healed.

But it was a temporary reprieve. At seventeen years of age, Savvy needed to have her temporomandibular joints (TMJs) replaced with custom titanium joints. They were worn out. We learned that joint damage was indeed systemic, as testing by Dr. Brendan Lee at Texas Children's and Baylor College of Medicine in Houston verified Hypermobile Ehlers-Danlos syndrome. Dr. Suresh Kotagal and Dr. Amir Orandi of Mayo Clinic Rochester also diagnosed POTS, medical PTSD, restless leg syndrome, and patella femoral disorder. The Daniel Amen Clinic SPECT exam verified a hypoxic brain injury.

What I know today, that was not known eighteen years ago when Dr. McKay's highly trained eye saw her at eighteen months, is that this was all **preventable**. Had Savvy been screened, evaluated, and treated before the age of six, she would not have had retractive orthodontic braces because she would not have needed them. Her jaws would have been gently and non-surgically brought forward by small, soft dental implements. Her upper palate would have been expanded together with her lower palate, all in an effort designed to ensure enough room for all thirty-two teeth to come in straight and ample space for her tongue to rest properly up and forward. Her nasopharynx complex would have been treated, too, and she would have learned to breathe through her nose and close her mouth.

James Nestor, a preeminent breathing expert and best-selling author, has underscored that no facet of our health is more vital than breathing. And yet, why didn't any of the medical professionals present at Savvy's birth recognize the potential impediment to her breathing and future development? "We see what we know" is an adage among experts. Tragically, over a span of nineteen years, the things they couldn't see of Savvy's condition precipitated a cascade of devastating injuries caused by oxygen deprivation and related comorbidities. A significant portion of these hardships could have been circumvented with early awareness and intervention, coupled with knowledge of airway disorders across all primary medical fields.

What if I had known then what I know now? That is the question I want to prevent you from asking yourself over and over. If only I had recognized the subtle signs earlier and taken action, perhaps her life would be different today, and we would have been saved from years of pain, heartache, and confusion. If I could turn back time, armed with the knowledge I have now, we could have spared Savvy years of suffering and loss, saved ourselves hundreds of thousands of dollars in search of answers, and spent the days and weeks of time used for research and traveling to various doctors differently, which is why it's so important that you are made aware of this silent pandemic.

So, I am sounding the alarm! There are almost two billion children on the planet. How are we going to help almost twenty percent of them when we now know that airway and sleep disorders are avoidable and treatable? If we can screen, evaluate, and treat them before they ever start school, their bodies will not feel like they are rotting, and their improved memories and concentration will give them the very start in life that every child deserves! Plus, society will not bear the cost of lost productivity caused by a lifetime of heart disease, diabetes, cognitive decline, and other conditions that can contribute to disability, joblessness, and abject poverty.

My journey as a mother and my personal experience with my daughter's airway disorder inspired me to establish the

Children's Airway First Foundation (CAFF). My hope is that no parent will have to navigate the complicated and distressing world of undiagnosed airway health disorders without assistance and knowledge. With this initiative, we're standing up against a silent pandemic, advocating for our children's health, and fighting to ensure that every child can breathe, sleep, and grow in the best possible way.

This book serves a dual purpose: first, to shine a light on the intricate realm of pediatric airway disorders through the lens of Savvy's harrowing journey, and second, to equip parents and caregivers with the knowledge to recognize risks, advocate for their child, and make informed decisions regarding their care.

This book is for the mothers who sense something is amiss but can't pinpoint it and the fathers baffled by their child's symptoms. It's for the caregivers searching for solutions and the healthcare providers seeking to treat the whole child. Through the sharing of our personal journey, I hope to help you learn and recognize the signs in your own child before it's too late and give you the tools and knowledge that I wish I had early on to advocate for them when needed.

This book will show you what to look for in your child and other children in your life of all age groups. Watch them sleep. Use our checklists. If needed, have them evaluated further with an airway-centric dentist or pediatrician. Learn to ask the right questions that will avoid misdiagnoses and help us all advocate for changes in medical and dental school curricula. It is estimated that only three percent of our medical schools teach primary care and pediatric physicians to diagnose and treat airway and sleep conditions. Many spend only four hours in medical school touching on this life-saving and life-changing knowledge. This is about all of us! It's about the kid next door and the child whose disabilities and inability to think clearly due to a hypoxic brain and body keep them from reaching his or her full potential. We all must help these kids! This is a true public health crisis, little known and under-recognized.

Our children's quality of life depends on us learning this information and advocating for them today.

ONE
AIRWAY HEALTH AND THE URGENCY OF NOW

Is your child breathing comfortably and effortlessly, both during the day and at night?

Checklist for Recognizing Signs of Airway Disorders:

<u>Physical Signs</u>

- Are your child's teeth misaligned or crowded?
- Does your child have an unusually high and narrow palate?
- Do they struggle with nasal congestion, particularly when sleeping?
- Are they prone to snoring and restless sleep?
- Does your child have a jaw that appears set back or underdeveloped?
- Have you noticed a narrowing or sinking of the upper facial features—lip, nose, or cheekbones?

- Is your child overweight, increasing their risk of sleep apnea?

Hidden Signs

- Does your child suffer from persistent allergies affecting their breathing?
- Are ear infections a recurring issue?
- Have you observed any delays in your child's speech development?

Emotional Signs

- Does your child show signs of mood swings or irritability?
- Are they less interactive or more withdrawn than usual?

Mental Signs

- Is it difficult for your child to focus, affecting school performance?
- Does your child seem unusually tired or lethargic during the day?
- Are there dark circles under their eyes, indicating sleep deprivation?

These questions are designed to guide your understanding of the multi-faceted nature of airway disorders but do not encompass all of the airway health-related evaluation questions. If you find yourself answering yes to multiple items on this checklist, it may be time to seek the expertise of healthcare professionals who can diagnose and manage airway health issues. But first, read on to learn more.

WHAT IS AIRWAY HEALTH? : "THE BREATH WE TAKE FOR GRANTED"

Every breath we draw should be a testament to the miracle of life. Yet, increasingly, these breaths have become labored, fraught with struggle, and many of us don't realize it because all we know is how we've always breathed. Airway health disorders are quietly wreaking havoc, becoming a silent pandemic that fails to make the headlines but invades our homes, affecting both young and old.

For my daughter, Savvy, mere moments after her birth, clues were present. A high V-shaped dental arch, lips with an accentuated cupid's bow indicative of improper muscle tone, and a flaccid lower lip that rolled outward—all classic signs of a mouth breather.

Airway health silently, yet profoundly, shapes children's well-being while most of us remain in the dark about its existence and effects. A critical reason for this lack of awareness is the tendency to normalize symptoms of airway disorders such as snoring and mouth breathing as harmless, transient quirks. In reality, these seemingly innocuous signs often mask a much larger, underlying health concern. Yet ninety-five percent of cases go undiagnosed, leaving ten to twelve percent of children habitually snoring, twenty-five percent of children chronically breathing through their mouth, and misdiagnoses, like ADHD, becoming common due to over-lapping symptoms.[1]

Pediatric airway problems can be likened to the struggle of breathing through a narrow straw. The effects span from mild symptoms like congestion to more serious conditions such as sleep disruption, oxygen deprivation, recurrent infections, and developmental delays in speech. The chronic stress brought on by these issues exacts a toll on both physical and mental health.

The airway, which refers to the passages that facilitate the flow of air to and from the lungs, forms an essential part of the respiratory system. It commences at the nose and mouth and facilitates the inhalation of oxygen and exhalation of carbon dioxide, contributing to our very survival. The upper airway comprises the nasal cavity, mouth, pharynx, and larynx, where structures filter, humidify, and regulate airflow. The lower airway, consisting of the trachea and bronchi, conducts air directly into the lungs.

The appropriate development of these structures is imperative for effective breathing. Any alteration in their anatomy, whether from birth or occurring later through improper development, can affect airway patency. Similarly, external influences like allergens, pollutants, and tobacco smoke also bear significant impact on airway function.

Airway health disorders are structural, systematic, genetic, and environmental.

When we talk about airway issues, let me be clear that we're not just discussing the immediate discomfort of a blocked nose or snoring. In children, these disorders are developmental detours with potentially long-term consequences. Speech delays, difficulties in concentration, behavioral issues, and even lowered academic performance can all be downstream effects of poor airway health.

As we age, the stakes get even higher. For adults, poor airway health isn't just an inconvenience; it's often a silent catalyst for a myriad of other health issues. Think about the toll that sleep apnea takes on the cardiovascular system or how chronic fatigue induced by poor sleep can lead to mental health issues like depression and anxiety. These aren't isolated problems but interconnected health challenges that can often be traced back to compromised airways.

SLEEPING AND BREATHING

"Every major system, tissue, and organ of your body suffers when sleep becomes short. No aspect of your health can retreat at the sign of sleep loss and escape unharmed. Like water from a burst pipe in your home, the effects of sleep deprivation will seep into every nook and cranny of biology, down into your cells, even altering your most fundamental self—your DNA."[2]

AN EXCERPT FROM *WHY WE SLEEP* BY
MATTHEW WALKER

If you are concerned that your child has an airway disorder or wondering if they do, one of the best first steps you can take is to watch them sleep.

When we consider a good night's sleep, it's not just about the quantity; the quality of sleep plays an equally critical role. That's where the health of our child's airway comes into focus.

Imagine your child lying down to rest after a long day full of learning and play. You might think that the moment their eyes close, their body switches off, but that's not the case. Sleep is an active process involving various stages, each contributing to restorative functions essential for their physical growth, cognitive development, emotional regulation, and overall health.

Now imagine if, during this vital process, their airway— the passage that allows for the free flow of air to their lungs— is compromised. This could be due to factors like enlarged tonsils or adenoids, allergies, or even craniofacial features like a receded jaw or a high-arched palate. This disruption could mean that with every breath your child takes, they're working harder to get the oxygen they need. This struggle, though they might not be consciously aware of it, can lead to interrupted sleep or lighter, less restful sleep stages.

The effects of poor-quality sleep due to airway disorders can show up in various, often subtle ways. Perhaps your child is constantly tired, even after what seems like a full night's sleep, or they have difficulty concentrating or are displaying behavioral issues. Maybe they're snoring, a sign often wrongly assumed as deep sleep, but it could be an indicator of a struggling airway. When we stayed in hotels, I would hear Savvy grinding her teeth, known as bruxism. She tossed and turned all night, waking up often as she tried to sleep.

Airway disorders, particularly when they disrupt sleep, are not just a nighttime issue. The consequences seep into the daytime, affecting their energy levels, learning abilities, mood, growth, and overall health. In short, the quality of your child's sleep can ripple out to affect the quality of their life.

UCLA neurologist Ron Harper's research highlights the dire impacts of childhood sleep disorders, linking sleep apnea to early brain damage. Extensive studies demonstrate these conditions' effects on developing brains. Simple tests can reveal problems with gray matter and prefrontal lobe function, though rarely performed.[3] A disconnect persists between research and clinical practice, causing children like Savvy needless harm.

Obstructive sleep apnea (OSA) is a sleep-related breathing disorder characterized by reduced or halted airflow despite ongoing efforts to breathe. This occurs when the muscles at the back of the throat fail to keep the airway open, regardless of breathing efforts. These episodes lead to decreases in blood oxygen levels, often coinciding with reduced blood oxygen saturation. These obstructions can result in abrupt awakenings from sleep to resume breathing—an event that the child might not consciously register. What parents do not realize is that when these episodes occur, it can be equated to your child choking and having their air supply cut off. If we knew that was happening on a regular basis, it may get our attention more so.

Children with OSA may exhibit symptoms distinct from adults. These symptoms can be broadly classified into nighttime and daytime symptoms.

Nighttime symptoms may include:

- Loud snoring punctuated by pauses, snorts, or gasps
- Restless sleep and abnormal sleeping positions
- Bedwetting (particularly if the child had previously established good nighttime bladder control)
- Profuse sweating during sleep
- Observed episodes of breathing difficulty or cessation during sleep
- Frequent nightmares or night terrors

Daytime symptoms may include:

- Morning headaches
- Excessive daytime sleepiness or lethargy
- Behavioral issues such as irritability, aggression, or hyperactivity
- Concentration difficulties or poor academic performance
- Slowed growth or failure to thrive

Obstructive breathing disorders are a common issue among children and affect millions globally. The prevalence varies, with conditions like OSA and asthma being particularly common in pediatric populations. The most prevalent cause of OSA in children is enlarged tonsils and adenoids, but factors such as obesity, family history, exposure to allergens or pollutants, and inherent airway abnormalities play a role in these disorders' development.

Mouth breathing, characterized by habitual breathing through the mouth instead of the nose, is a commonly overlooked issue that parents need to be mindful of. Nasal breathing, which involves breathing through the nose, is the natural and optimal breathing method for children. The nose plays a crucial role in conditioning and filtering the air we breathe, ensuring it is adequately warmed, humidified, and purified from harmful particles. Nasal breathing also facilitates the efficient exchange of oxygen and carbon dioxide, supports optimal lung function, and contributes to balanced oral and facial development.

Chronic mouth breathing can result in a host of detrimental effects on a child's health and development, including disturbed sleep, altered facial and dental growth, speech and language issues, numerous cavities, oral health problems, and reduced physical endurance. Recognizing the signs of mouth breathing, such as an open mouth posture, dry lips, snoring, and chronic nasal congestion, allows parents to address the root causes and seek necessary treatment.

The American Academy of Sleep Medicine (AASM) recommends that children six to twelve years of age should sleep nine to twelve hours per twenty-four hours. However, six out of ten children get less than nine hours. Teenagers aged thirteen to eighteen years of age should sleep eight to ten hours per twenty-four hours, while seven out of ten teens sleep less than eight hours.[4]

According to the CDC, insufficient sleep is a public health epidemic.[5] More than one-third of adults fail to obtain the recommended seven to nine hours of nightly sleep. The genetic characteristic BHLLE4, which enables a person to function well with only six hours of nightly sleep, is very rare, so for most of us, this limited amount of sleep is severely detrimental.

A momentary lapse in concentration is called a microsleep. During a microsleep, your brain becomes blind to the outside world for a brief moment in all channels of perception. My daughter's teacher reported Savvy's microsleeps to me when she was only ten years of age. They are usually suffered by individuals who are chronically sleep restricted, defined as getting less than seven hours of sleep per night on a routine basis.

Guess what? The shorter you sleep, the shorter your healthspan and lifespan. When you're awake for more than sixteen hours, your brain begins to fail. Routinely sleeping less than six hours per night weakens your immune system, substantially increases your risk of certain forms of cancer or Alzheimer's disease, disrupts blood sugar levels to prediabetic levels, and contributes to obesity and the likelihood of your coronary arteries becoming blocked and brittle, leading to cardiovascular disease, stroke, and congestive heart failure.

Data from the American Academy of Sleep Medicine indicates that 5.9 million U.S. adults are diagnosed with OSA, but a staggering 23.5 million remain undiagnosed.[6] Approximately ninety-five percent of children with OSA are never diagnosed. Undiagnosed and untreated sleep disorders have significant impacts on mental health and daily functioning.

The Patient-Centered Primary Care Collaborative (PCPC-C.org) reported in 2019 that sixty-five to ninety percent of adults with depression suffer from sleep disorders. It's worth noting that mental health issues don't exist in a vacuum; they often coexist with other medical conditions. When we think about the same data in relation to children, a similarly worrying pattern emerges. The PCPCC.org study also reported that twenty-five to fifty percent of children with ADHD suffer from sleep disorders.[7]

Dr. David Gozal, a pediatric pulmonologist and sleep medicine specialist, hammers home the seriousness of the situation by saying, "The quality of life of a child that has sleep apnea is equivalent to that of a child with cancer receiving chemotherapy."[8] Yet, the cruel twist of fate lies in our blindness towards the grave consequences of airway disorders. The struggle of a child with sleep apnea or persistent snoring is no less traumatic than the ordeal of chemotherapy, but it mostly remains unnoticed and undiagnosed.

In spite of extensive research and innumerable studies dedicated to children's sleep disorders and sleep medicine, society remains startlingly ill-equipped to confront the reality of these conditions. Therefore, as parents, it becomes crucial for us to remain vigilant about our children's sleep habits, such as mouth breathing, snoring, restlessness, frequent awakenings, daytime fatigue, or behavioral changes, and we can be proactive as early as when the child is in the womb.

TWO
THE MARVELS OF IN-UTERO DIAGNOSTICS

Over the past few years, since we started the Children's Airway First Foundation (CAFF) to help other parents and kids, we have learned that Savvy's airway could have been corrected as early as right after birth. When asked why Savvy's health continued to decline after the orthognathic surgery at thirteen, Dr. Hang suggested it was because the fire was lit in utero. She exhibited these traits from birth—she was a mouth breather, likely affecting her sucking in utero.

Dr. Deborah Krakow at UCLA is world-renowned for her work in skeletal dysplasia, maternal-fetal health, obstetrics and gynecology, orthopedics, and genetics. She did an ultrasound on my granddaughter at twenty-six weeks gestation. The hard palate was wide and healthy; the jaw alignment was perfect. Each measurement was perfect. Paying attention to these things is key while they're in the womb. Sometimes, the palate is too high and impedes nasal breathing since the roof of the mouth is the floor of the nasal cavity. Maybe the lower jaw, mandible, is retrognathic or retruded. There may be a tongue tie, which could cause the tongue to block the back of the throat and impair breathing.

It's absolutely vital to understand that science and medical technology have advanced to a stage where we can indeed identify signs of potential airway disorders while your baby is still in the womb.

This groundbreaking capability is more than just noteworthy; it's an urgent call to action that we must heed. For decades, ultrasound technology has been utilized for anatomical assessments and to monitor the growth of the fetus. Recent advancements in high-resolution ultrasound technology can now help us go beyond just measuring the length of a femur or looking at the shape of the skull. We can actually scrutinize the development of oral and facial structures and, in some cases, even catch early indicators of potential airway issues.

It's not just about catching a glimpse of your child during these ultrasound appointments. It's also about utilizing this technology as a proactive tool for health.

- Identification of Craniofacial Anomalies: The development of the baby's face, skull, and neck are closely monitored during ultrasound scans. Any potential issues, such as a cleft lip or palate or masses in the neck area, can potentially impact the baby's airway after birth.

- Nasal Bone Length: You might wonder, why the nose? Anomalies in nasal bone length are a critical clue and can be an early warning sign of airway obstruction. Abnormal nasal bone lengths have been linked to the risk of respiratory issues, including obstructive sleep apnea.

- Jaw Structure: The jaw isn't just for adorable baby smiles; it's the foundation of their airway. An underdeveloped or misaligned jaw may signal insufficient space for a proper airway, possibly leading to issues like sleep-disordered breathing.

- Fetal Movements: Movements of the fetus, particularly those of the mouth and diaphragm, provide valuable information about the development of the airway and breathing mechanisms. If there are abnormalities in these movements, this might suggest potential issues with the airway or nervous system.

- Amniotic Fluid Volume: Amniotic fluid is crucial for the development of the baby's lungs and airway. Too much or too little amniotic fluid can impact this development. An imbalance in amniotic fluid can also hint at issues with the baby's ability to swallow, which involves the same muscles as breathing.

- Growth Patterns: Growth restriction in utero could indicate an underlying issue that might affect the baby's overall development, including the development of the airway and respiratory system. Close monitoring of the baby's growth can help identify such issues.

All these potential issues can be picked up during regular prenatal care visits. The ultrasound is a powerful tool, not just for parents to see their baby but also for medical professionals to ensure the baby's healthy development. If a potential issue is identified, it can lead to a more detailed assessment, such as a fetal MRI, consultations with pediatric specialists, or even in-utero treatment in some cases.

Once we have this invaluable data, a specialized medical team—pediatricians, osteopaths, ENT specialists, and often orthodontists—can formulate a customized action plan. This isn't just about taking notes; this is about taking decisive, possibly life-changing action. We'll talk about what this looks like more in chapter nine.

Identifying these signs in utero isn't about labeling or stigmatizing your child with a condition before they're even born. It is about equipping yourself with invaluable knowledge that can guide preventative and early intervention strategies. Imagine being able to address these issues before your child takes their first breath at birth. Imagine setting them on a course toward optimal health from day one that you can be certain of. Isn't that what we all want for our children?

When it comes to airway health, the clock starts ticking long before a child takes their first breath. Diagnosing an issue in utero opens a window of opportunity, a precious timeframe within which intervention can radically improve a child's quality of life. We're talking about the difference between years of struggling and a future where every breath comes easily.

This isn't just about sidestepping immediate problems. This is about sidestepping a lifetime of struggles that can come with mismanaged airway health—struggles with attention, struggles with behavior, and yes, struggles with every breath. The chance to correct or even prevent these issues before they become lifelong challenges is not just a window of opportunity; it's a lifeline!

Let's be clear: detecting potential airway disorders in utero is not a guarantee that your child will face these issues. However, knowledge is power—the power to monitor, the power to prepare, and the power to act. This isn't just revolutionary; it's a call to action that we, as parents, healthcare providers, and a society invested in the well-being of our next generation, cannot afford to turn a deaf ear to.

With the advent of these extraordinary diagnostic tools, we have been handed the reins to take control of our children's health even before they enter the world. This is groundbreaking. This is monumental. This is an opportunity we can't afford to miss.

THREE
THE URGENCY OF MONITORING SLEEP AND BREATHING IN AGES 0-2

Do You Know How Your Child Sleeps?

- Is your baby excessively noisy or straining when breathing?
- Does your child frequently snore during sleep?
- Does your baby wake up multiple times in the night, often gasping or choking?
- Is your child experiencing difficulty with feeding?
- Is your baby often irritable and hard to settle?
- Have you noticed an open mouth breathing habit?
- Does your baby suffer from frequent respiratory infections?
- Is your child lagging behind in speech and motor skill development?
- Have you noticed any instances of breath-holding or seeming to forget to breathe?
- Does your baby have blue-tinged lips or skin, especially during sleep?

If you find yourself answering yes to any of these questions, don't let another breath go by without action. Consult a medical professional experienced in pediatric airway health. Early detection isn't just preventive; it's often life-changing.

A recurring issue that haunts me is the fact that children born with anatomical anomalies in their jaws and craniofacial respiratory complex, like Savvy, often fare the worst when it comes to airway disorders. Craniofacial respiratory complex includes the nasal cavity, oral cavity, pharynx (the cavity behind the nose and mouth that leads to the esophagus), larynx (voice box), and even the craniofacial bones and muscles that support these structures and enable their function, which work together to allow effective breathing.

The development, size, shape, and function of these components are critical for maintaining an open and effective airway. Alterations or abnormalities in any part of this complex, whether due to congenital factors, growth, or environmental influences (like mouth breathing or the use of pacifiers and bottles), can influence the overall functioning of the airway.

When Savvy was born, I noticed that the space between her upper lip and the bottom of her nose, often referred to as the philtrum, was too small. I brushed it off as a familial characteristic, not realizing that it was a sign of Savvy's future struggles.

The distance between the nose base and the upper lip can be significant because this region forms part of the nasal complex and oral structures, all of which are essential for a functioning airway. A smaller philtrum could be indicative of an overall reduced midface size or underdevelopment, which may result in a smaller nasal cavity or a narrow, high-arched palate.

The development of the midface is closely tied to the formation and growth of other structures like the jaw and the dental arch. Anomalies in this region might also be associated with other oral and maxillofacial irregularities like a receded or small jaw (micrognathia or retrognathia) or dental malocclusions, all of which can contribute to a compromised airway.

These conditions can affect the child's ability to breathe efficiently through their nose, causing them to become mouth breathers.

Airway disorders manifest themselves in multiple ways. Perhaps one of the most recognizable signs is the condition known as scalloping. This refers to the unusual imprint of the tongue on the sides of the teeth, indicating that the tongue is pressing against the teeth due to a lack of space or improper positioning. While scalloping is a clear sign of an airway issue, it is often overlooked by medical professionals due to insufficient training in recognizing it. Savvy was surrounded by the very best medical professionals from the beginning, but since no one was trained to spot airway disorders, they missed the physical signs in Savvy until it was too late.

This is why an airway health exam from the moment they're born is so important to be ready to do.

What Doctors Should Check:

- General Respiratory Function: Observing the baby's breathing patterns for signs of stridor, wheezing, or irregularities.
- Facial Structure: Checking for high-arched palates, narrow nasal passages, or other craniofacial features that could affect the airway.
- Lip and Tongue Ties: Assessing whether these tethered tissues are present and if they are affecting feeding or breathing.

- Nasal Patency: Ensuring the nasal passages are clear and not obstructed.
- Oxygen Saturation Levels: Some doctors recommend a pulse oximetry test to measure oxygen levels in the blood.
- Latch and Sucking Mechanisms: Especially important for breastfeeding babies, poor latching could indicate an issue.

I had the privilege of meeting Dr. Chelsea Pinto, an extraordinary dentist with a specialized focus on airway development for children from birth to age two. Initially part of the Breathe Institute with Dr. Zaghi in Los Angeles, she now runs her own practice in Woodland Hills. Dr. Pinto's focus on these early years is crucial, given that about ninety percent of brain development occurs before a child turns three. This makes proper oxygenation absolutely vital for cognitive growth.

Dr. Pinto's expertise proved particularly helpful in evaluating lip, buccal, and tongue ties, which I experienced first-hand with my month-old granddaughter. Medically known as ankyloglossia, tongue-tie is a condition present at birth that restricts the tongue's range of motion due to a short or tight frenulum—the band of tissue connecting the underside of the tongue to the floor of the mouth. The tongue plays a crucial role in swallowing, breathing, and oral cavity development. These ties can contribute to chronic mouth breathing, which lowers the oxygen levels reaching an infant's rapidly developing brain.

Lip and tongue ties can also hinder an infant's ability to latch onto a breast or bottle, leading to a failure to thrive due to inadequate nutrient intake. According to Dr. Suresh Kotagal, a pediatric neurologist and sleep specialist retired from the Mayo Clinic Rochester, the development of myelin and neurotransmitters is crucial in these early years for children and essential for the normal functioning of the human brain. Breast milk is the fuel for producing these.

Myelin is a fat-rich substance that encases nerve fibers and improves the speed and efficiency of nerve signal transmission. This process begins while a baby is still in the womb, continuing throughout childhood and even into their mid-twenties. Premature birth, before thirty-five weeks of gestation, can interrupt this critical development, possibly leading to challenges related to nerve function and communication later in life.[1]

Neurotransmitters, the brain's primary chemical messengers, facilitate communication between neurons. They play a vital role in numerous physiological functions, from triggering muscle movement to influencing mood. The skin-to-skin contact and eye contact that occur during breastfeeding stimulate brain development and the release of neurotransmitters like oxytocin. This hormone, known as the "love hormone," helps build the mother-infant bond and plays a significant role in brain development. The production and regulation of these chemicals start in the womb and extend into postnatal life. For example, myelination, the process of neurotransmitter production, can also be disrupted by premature birth, potentially impacting a child's future neurological and physiological health.

Breast milk is rich in nutrients, including proteins, fats, and complex carbohydrates, that are crucial for myelination and the overall growth of the brain. It also contains bioactive compounds that help with the production and function of neurotransmitters. Breastfeeding can provide protection against a variety of infections, including those of the respiratory tract, which may help maintain a clear airway and reduce the likelihood of breathing-related issues.

Breastfeeding also plays a profound role in shaping the

normal growth and function of a child's airway structures. The intricate motions of sucking, swallowing, and breathing during breastfeeding actively influence the development of the oral cavity, nasal airway, and facial muscles, all of which are critical for unobstructed breathing.

When a baby suckles at the breast, the tongue presses against the hard palate while the jaw and facial muscles generate a rhythmic sucking motion. This stimulation encourages normal development of the hard palate, promoting ample room for proper tongue position and preventing a high-arched, narrow palate that can obstruct airflow.

The strength and endurance required to extract milk, often over long feeding sessions, helps tone and train the muscles of the tongue, cheeks, lips, and jaw for optimal strength and mobility. These robust oral muscles are then able to maintain proper rest postures of the tongue and surrounding structures, keeping the airway open.

During breastfeeding, the infant coordinates breathing through the nose while feeding. This nasal breathing strengthens the nasal airway muscles and allows ideal airflow resistance to occur within the nose, encouraging its optimal growth and patency.

Research shows that breastfed infants have a lower incidence of breathing issues and fewer upper respiratory infections, likely conferred by the immune factors in human milk.[2] Breastfeeding is also associated with reduced overbite and improved facial symmetry compared to bottle feeding.[3]

My relationship with Savvy is especially close, partly due to my decision to breastfeed her until she was thirty-two months old—something quite rare nowadays—which kept her in my arms for the first part of her life. I had to stop breastfeeding due to a medical procedure that required me to be sedated. Merely weeks later, Savvy was hospitalized with RSV, marking the first time she had ever fallen ill.

The abrupt change in her health status was a shock to us. It felt like the end of breastfeeding opened the door to illness, something she'd never experienced before. Despite the fact that the emergency room at Seattle Children's Hospital was full of kids sick with RSV, it still felt unsettling due to her previously robust health. The sudden break from our established routine was undoubtedly traumatizing for her, yet she never cried or whined, adapting quickly to the changes.

"Many things can wait. Children cannot. Today their bones are being formed, their blood is being made, their senses are being developed. To them we cannot say 'tomorrow.'"

— *GABRIELA MISTRAL*

Monitoring for potential issues is about maintaining a keen eye on how your child breathes, sucks, and swallows. A baby's ability to breathe comfortably, latch onto the breast during feeding, and swallow milk effectively are all important indicators of their airway health. Unusual sounds, frequent interruptions in breathing, or difficulty with breastfeeding can all be red flags that signal potential problems.

It is true that recognizing normal from abnormal in newborn behavior can be challenging, especially for first-time parents. Not every baby who has trouble feeding or makes unusual noises has an airway disorder. However, knowing what to look for will help parents identify when to seek medical advice. Let's look at some of these indicators more closely:

- Breathing: It's normal for a baby to breathe rapidly, then slowly, then pause for up to five to ten seconds before starting again. This pattern is called periodic breathing, and it usually doesn't mean that the baby is having trouble breathing. However, if your baby's breathing is consistently fast (more than sixty breaths per minute) or slow (less than thirty breaths per minute), or if they have frequent, long pauses in their breathing, this could be a sign of an airway issue.

- Feeding: A healthy baby should be able to latch onto the breast or a bottle nipple comfortably and stay latched for a good amount of time to feed effectively. If your baby frequently unlatches, seems to struggle with staying latched, or is not gaining weight appropriately, this could indicate an issue with sucking or swallowing and could be related to an airway disorder.

- Noises: Some noises are normal for babies, such as grunts, gurgles, or sighs. However, high-pitched noises, especially during inhalation (stridor), can be a sign of an airway issue such as laryngomalacia or tracheomalacia. Persistent wheezing, frequent coughing, or other unusual sounds can also be red flags.

- Other signs: Other signs that your baby may have an airway disorder include persistent blue coloring around the lips and mouth (cyanosis), frequent choking or gagging (especially during feeds), and unusual head or neck postures. A baby who consistently arches their neck back during feeds may be doing so to open their airway.

If your baby shows any of these signs, it's important to consult with a healthcare professional. They can assess your baby's symptoms, perform necessary tests or imaging studies if needed, and provide guidance on the next steps.

Furthermore, it's essential to realize that while these are general guidelines, each child is unique, and what might be a sign of a problem in one child might not be in another. Trust your instincts—if something doesn't feel right, it's always worth getting it checked out.

OSTEOPATHS

In the early stages of a child's life, particularly from zero to two years, the adverse impacts of inadequate oxygenation could lead to long-lasting damage. Various professionals, from dentists to myofunctional therapists, often overlook this critical period, delaying intervention until thirty months to four years old for many medical areas. The only practitioners I found addressing these issues from infancy were osteopaths, who manually manipulate the upper palate and advance the jaw, which could be a game-changer. But how many parents know about osteopaths or are referred to them?

Osteopathy is a branch of healthcare that emphasizes the role of the musculoskeletal system in health and disease. Osteopaths take a holistic approach to healthcare, under-standing that all parts of the body are interconnected. They use manual techniques to balance all the body systems, improving overall health and well-being. For infants with airway disorders, an osteopath may use gentle manipulation to improve the function and alignment of the bones, muscles, and connective tissue in and around the airway. Osteopaths also provide guidance on exercises and techniques that parents can use at home to support their baby's development and overall health. This may include exercises to help the baby open their mouth wider or strategies to improve tongue mobility and strength.

Moreover, osteopaths can play an essential role in the early detection of potential airway disorders. They are trained to observe and understand the subtle signs of these conditions, often before they become more apparent or problematic. Early detection and intervention, as we've discussed, can significantly improve long-term outcomes.

When Savvy was all wired up for surgery at the age of thirteen, she was in so much discomfort. A renowned myofunctional therapist, Joy Moeller, recommended we take her to an osteopath, so we found one. He looked over at Savvy and said, "I'm sorry, there's nothing I can do. If I had seen her as a child, I would have changed the shape of her palate and moved her jaw forward manually. I could have made those adjustments for her as a child, but now it's too late."

If I could do it again, I would have an osteopath in the room the moment Savvy was delivered, which is why it's so crucial we educate expectant mothers about these issues. The fear of damage to their child's brain is likely to motivate them to seek early intervention. Savvy's journey is a testament to this.

The importance of early detection and intervention becomes abundantly clear when we consider the immediate benefits that it brings. When an airway disorder is identified at an early stage, the window for effective intervention opens up. Early treatments help alleviate symptoms, leading to a significant improvement in a child's day-to-day life.

Imagine your child, who has been struggling with restless sleep due to an undiagnosed airway disorder, finally getting a good night's sleep. This would dramatically enhance their ability to concentrate and improve their overall behavior and mood. There would be noticeable improvements in their academic performance and the way they interact with their peers. In essence, the child who was previously struggling is now given the tools to thrive thanks to early intervention.

Looking beyond the immediate benefits, early intervention also prevents the development of more serious health conditions in the long run. Untreated airway disorders contribute to conditions like obesity, cardiovascular disease, and metabolic disorders. These are not minor complications but serious health conditions that can adversely affect an individual's quality of life.

DR. KAREN PARKER DAVIDSON - MESSAGE TO THE READER
4-PHASE RHINOMANOMETRY

By Dr. Karen Parker Davidson, MSA, M.Ed., MSN, RN

4-PHASE RHINOMANOMETRY IN THE PEDIATRIC POPULATION

The assessment of nasal function in children is crucial for early detection of respiratory issues that can impact their overall health. One of the most advanced methods for evaluating nasal airflow and resistance is 4-phase rhinomanometry (4PR). This non-invasive diagnostic tool provides comprehensive insights into the dynamics of nasal breathing across different phases of the respiratory cycle, making it particularly useful in pediatric populations where nasal obstruction and other functional issues often go unnoticed. Early detection of these problems is critical because impaired nasal function can affect not just breathing, but sleep quality, cognitive development, and overall body function.

UNDERSTANDING 4-PHASE RHINOMANOMETRY

4-phase rhinomanometry is a quick, non-invasive test that measures the pressure and airflow in both nostrils for 15 seconds during four key phases of the respiratory cycle: inspiration, expiration, and the transition phases between them. Unlike traditional rhinometry or x-rays, which provide a static assessment, 4PR allows for a dynamic evaluation of how air moves through the nasal passages during each breath. By capturing data on how much air resistance occurs during each phase, clinicians can pinpoint the level of resistance causing obstructions, asymmetries between the nostrils, or other issues affecting nasal patency.

In children, the nasal passages are smaller and more sensitive to inflammation or obstruction, making early detection of abnormalities crucial. In Japan and Europe, most children get their first baseline test at three years old. The studies found this can be done with high reliability and reproducibility. This is especially important as we can see dental changes at the age of two-to-three years old, and that is why we have a campaign, "We Can See At 3," to promote early testing in North America. 4PR offers a non-invasive, real-time assessment that can be easily tolerated by children, allowing for accurate diagnosis of conditions like allergic rhinitis, deviated septum, or enlarged adenoids. With this information, clinicians can intervene early, preventing long-term complications that could affect a child's development and quality of life.

4-phase rhinomanometry is a powerful tool for assessing nasal function in children, providing detailed and dynamic information about airflow resistance and breathing patterns. Early detection of nasal obstruction or dysfunction is critical, as these issues can lead to a range of complications, from sleep disturbances to cognitive impairments. By using 4PR, clinicians can identify nasal problems early and initiate treatment, ensuring that children develop healthy breathing habits that support their total body function, restful sleep, and optimal cognitive development. As such, the use of 4-phase rhinomanometry in pediatric care is not just a diagnostic tool but an essential part of comprehensive child health monitoring.

FOUR
UNVEILING THE HIDDEN SIGNS FOR AGES 3-5

Do You Know How Your Child Breathes?

- Does your child breathe primarily through their mouth, even when not exerting themselves?
- Is your child still snoring, or has snoring become more frequent?
- Have you noticed frequent pauses in breathing during sleep, followed by a gasp or a snort?
- Have you noticed frequent nighttime waking or restlessness?
- Do they struggle with persistent dark circles under their eyes?
- Are there recurrent bouts of night sweats?
- Have they experienced speech delays or difficulties?
- Do they exhibit recurrent mood swings, irritability, or aggressive behavior?
- Are they facing concentration issues or hyperactivity?

- Does your child suffer from regular ear infections or sinus issues?
- Have you observed a frequent forward head posture?

If you've ticked off any of these boxes, it may be time to consult with healthcare professionals experienced in airway health.

For many parents, the first few years of their child's life are a whirlwind of milestones and precious moments. Yet, it's within these formative years, specifically ages three to five, that crucial signs can appear. Airway health plays an understated but powerful role in shaping not only their physical features but also their emotional well-being and cognitive abilities. Early diagnosis isn't just proactive; it's protective. The global community is now waking up to its importance.

Renowned for his groundbreaking work in airway health, Dr. Jiro Abe has implemented programs in Japanese preschools aimed at early detection and intervention. He poses the question, "How can I get these toddlers fixed so that they can learn while they're in school?" His initiatives get every young child into curriculum-taught classes, turning myofunctional therapy exercises into fun and games.

Myofunctional therapy is a hidden gem of airway disorder treatment. This non-invasive approach focuses on retraining the facial and oral muscles to correct dysfunctional breathing patterns, swallowing, and tongue positioning. Trained therapists create individualized exercise regimens to improve muscle coordination and tone, optimizing airway function. Particularly effective for issues like mouth breathing, snoring, and sleep apnea, myofunctional therapy has garnered scientific backing, showing significant improvements in sleep quality and reductions in symptoms of airway disorders. For children, early intervention through this therapy can not only correct aberrant breathing habits but also positively influence facial development and even speech. The benefits aren't confined to younger populations; adults also report seeing enhancements in sleep quality and overall well-being after undergoing this treatment. With its focus on muscle function to facilitate easier breathing, myofunctional therapy offers a compelling, evidence-based avenue for those struggling with airway health issues, making it an essential part of a holistic approach to airway well-being.

By introducing these exercises focused on muscle function to facilitate easier breathing for kids at an early age, it opens up the door for correction while forming better habits and patterns that will continue to benefit them through adulthood. Dr. Abe offers essential training for teachers and parents, providing the tools to recognize and address airway disorders before they escalate.

Dr. Jeevanan Jahendran (Dr. J.J.), M.S. ORL, an ENT in Malaysia, said, "When a new patient walks into my practice, the first thing I look at is their gait!" You heard that right. It's not their ears, nose, and throat, as you may assume, but their gait! Savvy has flat feet, and I noticed her gait was changing when she was about four years of age.

Dr. J.J.'s approach speaks to the interconnectedness of the human body and the many subtle indicators that signal an underlying disorder. Dr. J.J.'s focus on gait rather than more overt symptoms like snoring or breathing difficulties is an innovative way to identify potential airway health problems. But how exactly can gait and airway health be related?

A person's gait can reveal a great deal about their overall health, including the alignment of their skeletal system, muscle function, and neurological condition. An abnormal gait may indicate that someone is compensating for discomfort or pain, which could be caused by any number of factors affecting the way they carry themselves. Someone who struggles with daytime fatigue because of an airway disorder may walk sluggishly or with less coordination. Flat feet, like in Savvy's case, can impact how one walks and may be correlated with changes in posture and alignment.

As we've discussed, airway disorders often compromise breathing, particularly during sleep, leading to conditions like sleep apnea. This disrupted sleep prompts the body to engage in compensatory behaviors—alterations in posture or walking patterns—as it seeks to adapt to reduced air intake. Over time, these compensatory changes impact musculoskeletal alignment, including foot posture, further weakening foot muscles needed to support the arch adequately, potentially contributing to Savvy's flat feet.

In contrast, most doctors are not trained to look for these unconventional signs of airway health disorders. Traditional medical training often emphasizes specialized knowledge— ENTs focus on the ears, nose, and throat; podiatrists look at the feet, and so on. Dr. J.J.'s approach, which brings a more holistic perspective to medical diagnosis, points to a broader understanding of how interconnected the body's systems truly are, which we'll dive more into in chapter eight.

Recognizing the relationship between gait and airway health adds another layer to diagnostic techniques and potentially leads to earlier, more effective interventions. However, it's worth noting that this is still a relatively unconventional and understudied approach, and more research is needed to conclusively link gait abnormalities to airway disorders. Dr. J.J.'s practice could serve as a starting point for more comprehensive studies in this fascinating interdisciplinary field.

Another cutting-edge diagnostic test that's rising is facial recognition technology, which is creating a new frontier for early, non-invasive, and data-driven medical interventions. Unlike traditional diagnostic methods that often involve lengthy and sometimes uncomfortable tests, facial recognition software analyzes subtle changes in facial structures indicative of disorders like sleep apnea, deviated septum, or chronic sinusitis within seconds. By comparing a patient's facial data to an extensive database of previously diagnosed cases, it holds the potential to identify risk factors long before conventional diagnostics would. This early detection not only facilitates quicker medical interventions but also optimizes the overall use of resources. The result? Patients have the opportunity to improve their quality of life sooner and at a reduced cost, as early detection usually entails less invasive and less expensive treatments.

Beyond its time and cost efficiency, facial recognition offers a distinct advantage in being non-invasive. Anyone who has gone through endoscopies or overnight sleep studies can attest to the discomfort and anxiety these tests can generate. However, a simple scan of a person's face eliminates these hardships, making the technology especially advantageous for children and those with sensitivities to medical procedures. It integrates seamlessly into routine check-ups without causing any discomfort, thereby reducing the risks associated with invasive diagnostic procedures.

Where facial recognition truly shines is in its data-driven approach. As algorithms continuously refine and update with new data, the technology promises an increasing reliability of diagnoses over time. It allows for the personalization of medical interventions by incorporating a wide array of variables, such as age, gender, and previous medical history, providing a more comprehensive understanding of an individual's condition.

Although the potential of facial recognition technology in

healthcare is substantial, it is not yet used. Rigorous clinical trials and ongoing research are essential steps toward validating its efficacy and ethical implications in a medical setting. However, it's important to know that this is in the works and to stay aware of any developments you hear about in relation to it.

In our journey with Savvy, our focus has been mainly on airway and sleep issues, but feedback from Texas Dell Children's Hospital pointed out that there could be other reasons for mouth breathing beyond structural anomalies. One such reason is severe allergies, which clog up nasal passages, preventing proper breathing and impacting sleep quality.

In a healthy airway, air moves freely, allowing your child to breathe without difficulty. Allergies can be a silent, yet significant, factor in children's airway health disorders, affecting a child's ability to breathe, swallow, and, ultimately, grow. Allergens such as pollen, dust mites, or pet dander can cause an overreaction in your child's immune system, leading to inflammation and swelling of the nasal passages and throat. This inflammation restricts air movement, causing symptoms such as snoring, mouth breathing, and restless sleep, which are all too often mistaken as mere nuisances rather than signs of a deeper issue.

A study published in *The Journal of Pediatrics* reports that children with allergic rhinitis, commonly known as hay fever, have a higher prevalence of sleep-disordered breathing. These children are also at a greater risk of developing obstructive sleep apnea, a severe form of this airway disorder [1].

As parents, recognizing the potential implications of allergies on your child's airway health is the first step toward a solution. Creating an allergen-free environment as much as possible is the next step. Regular cleaning, using air purifiers, and avoiding allergen triggers help reduce the severity of allergic reactions.

To limit exposure to allergens, the top suggestions are vacuuming every day and installing an air cleaner in a baby's room and around the house. These ideas resonated with me because my eldest son suffered from severe allergies. We had to move houses when he was a couple of years old and installed a new HVAC system equipped with HEPA filters to alleviate his constant discomfort. It was a trying time as he couldn't sleep, and the strong inhalers prescribed to him only increased his hyperactivity. Yet, no one informed us that it didn't have to be this way. The doctor insisted that his symptoms would dissipate with time, even though the inhaler made him shaky, which a five-year-old should not have to endure.

To ensure the well-being of our forthcoming granddaughter, we are creating a space in Savvy's house that will be vacuumed regularly and fitted with an air filter. We're taking extensive precautions, even down to the clothes worn in the room, to avoid potential allergens. Savvy didn't have such problems, possibly because I breastfed her for thirty-two months, which boosted her immune system. It wasn't until she was eight years old and exposed to cedar trees in Texas that she developed allergies. We are focused on preparing adequately to minimize the chances of our granddaughter developing any airway conditions.

A proactive approach, however, involves more than just symptom management. Regular check-ups with an allergist and a pediatric pulmonologist can help with monitoring your child's health, adjusting treatment plans as necessary. Early intervention and a tailored treatment plan can help ensure that your child's allergies do not stand in the way.

As a child grows into this stage, there are other signs to look out for. It's about observing more than just the physical symptoms. Behavioral issues can often be indicative of underlying health issues. Being aware of these signs can help you take action at the right time, setting the stage for effective intervention.

- Snoring: While occasional snoring is common, habitual snoring can be a sign of OSA. Research published in *Sleep Medicine Reviews* found that around ten percent of children are habitual snorers, and among them, approximately two to four percent have OSA.[1]

- Mouth Breathing: Healthy children typically breathe through their noses. Chronic mouth breathing can lead to abnormal facial growth, dental abnormalities, and poor sleep quality, among other issues. Mouth breathing can be indicative of various conditions such as adenoid hypertrophy, allergies, or nasal obstruction.[2]

- Restless Sleep: Restlessness during sleep, such as frequent tossing and turning, might indicate poor sleep quality, often related to sleep-disordered breathing conditions. The American Academy of Sleep Medicine points out that sleep disruptions caused by airway problems can lead to fragmented and non-refreshing sleep.[3]

- Recurring Ear and Sinus Infections: Frequent ear and sinus infections could point to an issue with the adenoids, which are part of the immune system and located near the airway. Enlarged adenoids have been associated with various airway problems.[4]

- Excessive Daytime Sleepiness: Excessive daytime sleepiness in children might suggest poor sleep quality or quantity at night, which could be due to an underlying sleep or airway disorder.

- Difficulty Concentrating and Hyperactivity: Children with sleep disorders may exhibit problems with attention, hyperactivity, and impulsivity. The American Academy of Pediatrics supports the correlation between sleep disorders and ADHD symptoms, citing that up to twenty-five percent of children with ADHD have sleep-disordered breathing.[5]

- Bedwetting: Sometimes, bedwetting can be a sign of OSA. Children with OSA may experience an increase in urine production during the night, which can lead to bedwetting.

- Frequent Nightmares or Night Terrors: Children experiencing interrupted sleep due to breathing issues may also have an increased likelihood of nightmares or night terrors.

- Delayed Growth or Failure to Thrive: Poor sleep quality or quantity due to airway disorders can affect a child's growth. As per a study in the *Journal of Clinical Sleep Medicine*, children with OSA often experience growth issues, potentially due to the energy expenditure of labored breathing or disruption in growth hormone production and release, which mainly happens during sleep.[6]

- Changes in School Performance: Sleep is critical for cognitive functions, including memory and attention. A decline in school performance might be indicative of a sleep disorder.

- Irritability or Mood Swings: Sleep deprivation caused by sleep disorders can lead to mood swings, irritability, or even depressive symptoms in children. Children with chronic sleep disorders often exhibit mood and behavioral issues.

- Frequent Headaches: Particularly morning headaches can be a symptom of sleep-disordered breathing. A study in the *Journal of Headache and Pain* found a significant association between morning headaches and sleep-disordered breathing in children and adolescents.[7]

- Overweight or Obesity: There's a complex relationship between sleep, metabolism, and weight. Sleep disorders, particularly sleep apnea, are more common in children with obesity.

Dr. Kevin Boyd points out that excessive cavities by the age of six could also indicate an airway disorder due to excessive mouth breathing. Before her orthognathic surgery, Savvy had twelve cavities that had never been identified or repaired.

Identifying these signs early and seeking professional advice can lead to effective interventions such as changes in a child's environment, medical treatments, or, in some cases, surgery. Additionally, in certain situations, a referral to a sleep specialist for a sleep study, or polysomnography, might be recommended.

Appropriate sleep testing is key in diagnosing and treating sleep disorders in children. Dr. Christian Guilleminault, a pioneer in the field of sleep medicine, recognized that sleep disorders in children, particularly obstructive sleep apnea, often showed up differently than in adults.

In adults, a polysomnogram (a type of sleep study) is typically used to identify sleep apnea. The standard threshold or cutoff point used to diagnose sleep apnea is typically five or more events of paused or shallow breathing per hour of sleep. This metric, known as the Apnea-Hypopnea Index (AHI), is widely accepted as a reliable measure for diagnosing sleep apnea in adults.

However, Dr. Guilleminault realized that this adult-based threshold was not adequately capturing sleep disorders in children. He saw children suffering from significant cognitive, behavioral, and growth issues related to disturbed sleep who didn't meet the adult AHI threshold. This led him to a game-changing revelation: children are not merely small adults, and they require a different diagnostic approach for sleep disorders.

Proposing a lower diagnostic threshold, Dr. Guilleminault argued that even one to three events of paused or shallow breathing per hour of sleep could indicate a problem in children. This was a substantial departure from the standard adult-focused AHI, highlighting the vulnerability of children to even mild disturbances in sleep.

In addition to altering the AHI, Dr. Guilleminault championed the inclusion of additional measurements in the routine sleep study protocol for children. These included tracking changes in esophageal pressure, monitoring oxygen and carbon dioxide levels, and examining the facial and craniofacial structures, which are pivotal in detecting subtle signs of sleep-disordered breathing in children. His work has emphasized that children have unique sleep needs, and a correct diagnosis must be based on their distinct characteristics, not merely an adaptation of adult standards. This paradigm shift has not only improved the precision of diagnosis but also led to more effective interventions, changing the lives of count-less children suffering from sleep disorders.

We'll talk more in chapter eight about these additional assessments and tools that may be used to diagnose and treat sleep disorders.

FIVE

NAVIGATING AIRWAY HEALTH FOR AGES 5-10

Have You Noticed Changes in Your Child's Smile?

- Does your child continue to snore loudly more nights than not?
- Is your child constantly tired, despite getting enough sleep?
- Are there instances of bedwetting?
- Has your child been diagnosed with ADD or ADHD?
- Does your child frequently complain of headaches or migraines?
- Is your child falling behind academically?
- Have you noticed frequent throat clearing or a persistent cough?
- Does your child struggle with poor dental health or malocclusion (misaligned teeth)?
- Is your child prone to anxiety or mood swings?
- Are there visible signs of chest retractions, especially when your child is exerting themselves?

If you find yourself worryingly ticking off multiple boxes on this list, it's high time you consult an expert in pediatric airway health. Don't let these formative years be choked by the invisible grip of airway disorders. Every breath counts when it comes to building a healthier, happier future for your child.

From ages five to eight, baby teeth make way for their adult successors, a phase most parents identify with photo album smiles and tooth fairy visits. But did you know that these years offer invaluable insight into your child's airway health? What can your child's emerging secondary teeth tell you about their well-being?

This stage is more than just a dental rite of passage; it's a crucial window for assessing and influencing airway health.

At eight years old, we moved to Austin, Texas. Savvy was accepted into one of the top private prep schools. The kids there start going, "Oh my God, look at those teeth!" Despite her intelligence and good heart, Savvy felt like the other kids didn't take the time to get to know her because of how she looked.

Savvy had an almost cartoonish grin, resulting from what I later learned was called a severe class II malocclusion, or a significant misalignment of teeth when the jaws are closed. She could not, and never could, close her mouth. It is what most of us may shrug off as a child who will grow into their mouth or who may need braces instead of recognizing it for the warning it is. However, it's a condition that dental experts will tell you never improves on its own. It requires intervention, including palatal expansion and jaw advancement. If not treated properly, the effects will compound throughout time.

There are four observable characteristics that pediatric professionals should look for to identify airway obstruction and disorders in children:

1. Class II Malocclusion: This refers to an overbite where the upper jaw and teeth significantly overlap the lower jaw and teeth. It is associated with airway issues because it may indicate a jaw structure that doesn't adequately support the airway.
2. Class III Malocclusion: Also known as an underbite, Class III malocclusion involves the lower jaw protruding beyond the upper jaw. While less commonly associated with airway issues than Class II, it can still indicate potential problems.
3. High V-Shaped Arch in Hard Palate: A high-arched palate reduces the volume of the nasal cavity and leads to a constricted airway, making breathing more laborious, especially during sleep.
4. Shortened Distance from Front to Back of Oral Cavity: A reduced space in the oral cavity could indicate a tongue that sits too far back, potentially causing obstruction of the airway.

Surprisingly, ninety-five percent of modern humans have deviations in dental alignment, and of that, thirty percent are recommended to have orthodontic treatment and fifty percent are recommended to have wisdom teeth removed. Worldwide prevalence of malocclusion among children and adolescents is fifty-six percent. Over ninety percent of children with crooked teeth, teeth grinding, or malocclusion have compromised nasal breathing.[1]

Knowing the evolutionary journey of our facial and dental structures and the impact it has is what will make us understand why this is so prevalent today. The transformation, which has been shaped by changes in our diets and lifestyles, profoundly affects not just our appearance but also the very functioning of our bodies. The shift from hunter-gatherer diets through farming and on to industrialized societies has left indelible marks on our facial morphology.

Our early ancestors, robust beings like Australopithecus, had large, protruding jaws reinforced by powerful muscles, designed to cope with a diet of tough, fibrous plants and raw meat. Chewing such food required considerable effort, which in turn demanded broader, flatter teeth, perfect for grinding. This strenuous lifestyle even influenced our nasal structures, leading to larger sinuses that could potentially warm and humidify the air, aiding efficient breathing during physical exertion.

Fast forward to the Agricultural Revolution; our dietary habits underwent a drastic change. People began to consume softer, processed foods such as grains and dairy products. This diet required less jaw power, and, over generations, our jaws and teeth adjusted accordingly. They became smaller, less robust, while our teeth became crowded—a testament to a gentler diet and a shrinking jaw.

Now in our modern industrialized era, with a plethora of processed, soft foods at our fingertips, the evolution continues. Our jaws are reducing in size, often leading to crowded teeth and malocclusion. Our faces are less pronounced, less rugged, with diminished brow ridges and smaller teeth. In fact, the potential impact of contemporary practices like bottle-feeding, pacifier use, and thumb-sucking on our infants' facial development is a hot topic of research today.

The problem arises when these changes in our craniofacial structures aren't merely aesthetic. They have consequences that affect the health of our children. As our jaws shrink, the conditions known as micrognathia and retrognathia, characterized by undersized or receded jaws, become more common. These changes lead to a smaller oral cavity and a narrower airway, potentially causing breathing difficulties, particularly during sleep, which is why we are seeing an influx in health problems for children as well as adults.

Similarly, a high-arched or narrow palate, impacted some-times in the womb but also by habits like thumb sucking, bottle-feeding, or consuming a soft diet, can also lead to a constricted airway, posing risks of sleep apnea or chronic mouth breathing.

And let's not forget the essential role of the tongue in maintaining an open airway.

In the proper resting position, the tongue should lie along the roof of the mouth, or palate, lightly touching the spot just behind the upper front teeth. The main body of the tongue should rest against the hard palate (the front part of the roof of the mouth). This position helps maintain an open space in the oropharynx, contributing to better airway patency. The back of the tongue should be elevated against the soft palate (the back part of the roof of the mouth), but without creating a sense of strain or blockage in the airway.

This tongue-to-palate resting position encourages nasal breathing and supports the proper development and align-ment of the teeth and jaws. Incorrect tongue posture, such as a low resting position of the tongue or tongue thrusting, also contribute to dental and craniofacial issues.

In our quest for the best orthodontic care for Savvy when she was eight years old, we sought the services of a top-rated local orthodontist based in Austin, Texas. It was his profes-sional opinion that Savvy would need double jaw surgery, medically known as orthognathic surgery (MMA). This, however, would have to wait until she was at least seventeen years old due to the developmental concerns associated with performing such a procedure at her tender age. In the interim, the orthodontist suggested a temporary measure: orthodontic braces, a path that is very normalized in today's age.

The plan entailed the use of a rapid expander on her

upper palate and retractive braces on her teeth to create a
visually appealing smile. We wanted Savvy to feel comfort-
able and confident, fitting in with her peers, so we agreed to
the plan. We had a series of appointments for regular adjustments over the subsequent months.

It was only many years later that I learned that even the
loss of a few millimeters of space in the mouth caused by the
retractive forces of braces can cause the tongue to be forced
further back into the throat. Retractive braces also often
necessitate the extraction of permanent teeth to make room
for realignment. This approach can be particularly detrimental in children with compromised airways, as the
resulting reduction in oral space further restricts proper
airflow and exacerbates existing breathing difficulties. This
displacement also indirectly affects nasal breathing by
changing the jaw's position, leading to increased nasal resistance. This nasal obstruction often results in a reliance on
mouth breathing, which further worsens airway-related
symptoms.

In children suffering from pre-existing airway disorders,
such as obstructive sleep apnea or chronic snoring, the symptoms might worsen when retractive braces treatment is initi-
ated or, even worse, when teeth are extracted. The resulting
changes can make the oral cavity smaller, resulting in further
airway collapse during sleep, increased episodes of apnea,
snoring, and disrupted sleep patterns.

The retractive forces exerted by braces can stress the
temporomandibular joint, which connects the jawbone to the
skull. In children with airway disorders, there might already
be an increased risk of TMJ dysfunction, and retractive braces
can further aggravate this condition, causing jaw pain,
clicking or popping sounds, headaches, and limited jaw
movement.

Knowing this, parents, it's vital that prior to initiating

orthodontic treatment, a thorough evaluation of a child's airway health is conducted. The potential impact of retractive braces on airway disorders can vary among individuals due to factors such as genetic predisposition, pre-existing anatomical variations, and the specific treatment plan. This assessment may involve an examination of the child's breathing patterns, sleep quality, nasal patency, and a screening for sleep-disordered breathing symptoms.

Recognizing and addressing underlying airway issues before orthodontic intervention can help mitigate potential risks. Therefore, orthodontic treatment plans should be personalized. In such cases, there should be a close collaboration among dentists, orthodontists, and sleep medicine specialists to ensure a comprehensive approach to treatment planning. This integrated approach allows for the inclusion of airway-focused treatment modalities such as myofunctional therapy, nasal breathing training, and orthodontic techniques that support optimal airway function, which we'll talk more about in chapter seven.

Unfortunately for us, we didn't realize the impact of the retractive braces on Savvy because we weren't aware of the conditions that already existed in her until it was too late.

Immediately after fitting her with the retractive braces and upper palate expander, we noticed a marked deterioration in her physical condition. This once energetic child who loved racing and exploring museums, who could sprint faster than anyone on the track, could no longer walk a short city block or run up the stairs to her favorite dinosaur exhibit at the Museum of Natural History without catching her breath. She had lost her stamina and started to gain weight.

Approximately a year following the removal of Savvy's expander and retractive orthodontics, her once captivating smile began to be overshadowed by an alarming concern. She began collapsing with physical exertion. At her school's fitness day celebration, she collapsed on the floor, gasping for air, after trying to jump rope for a minute. She was humiliated and embarrassed. Later, during a relay race, she collapsed again. We immediately took her to her new pediatrician in Austin, who diagnosed her with exercise-induced asthma, a condition where physical exertion triggers asthma symptoms. He prescribed inhalers and recommended a run-walk routine several times a week, along with advice on managing her allergy to cedar trees. Yet, the symptoms didn't completely align.

We never associated the changes with her orthodontic treatment until later. The decrease in her physical abilities, coupled with her previous confessions about feeling rotten and not as smart as before, were indicators of the harm inflicted on her due to the lack of proper oxygenation. Her struggles were akin to those of a child battling cancer, and yet we didn't see it because the harm was not as apparent.

In the fourth grade, Savvy developed a passion for volleyball. However, despite her enthusiasm, she faced obstacles due to frequent ankle injuries.

During this time, our consultations with her long-standing pediatrician were frustrating. His examination remained limited to his routine check-ups and did not extend to potential abnormalities. Even though Savvy repeatedly sprained her ankles, he did not evaluate the formation of her feet and knees or investigate potential skeletal issues. He noticed there were other signs—her scalloped tongue, worn teeth from grinding, and a tendency towards mouth breathing—but didn't know that they indicated a different underlying issue. Had the partially blocked airway been recognized and understood as being linked with her symptoms, we could have implemented necessary interventions much earlier. This oversight left us in the dark about Savvy's true health condition.

Our concerns escalated during a family trip to Sweden. As

we maneuvered through the airport, Savvy struggled to keep up with us. With her knees abnormally developing and signs of mouth breathing, exhaustion, brain fog, anxiety, and growing depression becoming more noticeable, it was evident that her health issues were intensifying.

Airway dysfunction can significantly impact energy levels and movement due to the oxygen that's crucial for generating energy within our cells. When the airway is obstructed or compromised, less oxygen reaches the lungs and, subsequently, less oxygen is delivered to the tissues and cells of the body. This results in lower energy production in the body, leading to fatigue and diminished stamina. For a child like Savvy, who was once full of energy, this meant a drastic reduction in her physical capabilities, such as walking a block or running up stairs without feeling winded.

In relation to movement, airway dysfunction interferes with the muscles' ability to function optimally. Reduced oxygen delivery to the muscles can lead to quicker exhaustion during physical activities, impacting overall performance. This was evident in Savvy's struggles with physical exertion, from her decreased athletic performance to her frequent ankle sprains. The frequent sprains could have been a result of her muscles tiring quickly due to decreased oxygenation, making them more susceptible to injury.

In Savvy's case, her endothelial system was not carrying enough oxygen in the blood to her muscles, and she had a collagen issue where those muscles could not support her joints. It changed her feet, her knees, her hips, and her entire growth. Then, when you add the retractive braces, it makes it worse and accelerates the process of dysplasias.

This reduction in oxygen supply also affects the brain, which relies heavily on oxygen for its functions. With less oxygen reaching the brain, symptoms such as brain fog, inability to concentrate, anxiety, and depression can manifest.

In Savvy's case, she noticed feeling less sharp or smart as before, a likely outcome of decreased oxygenation to her brain.

We took Savvy to Texas Children's in Houston, hoping to find answers we weren't getting in Austin. They ran tests. They took images. They told Savvy she was a mystery and should probably consider not going to such a stressful school anymore. Then they prescribed stronger inhalers and advised her to reduce stress, but, like her pediatrician, they failed to examine her knees, feet, and skeletal development. However, they did mention that she was using only forty-one percent of her lung capacity, a glaring red flag that was not investigated further.

We thought Savvy would like a break from school, so we took her with us on a business trip to China. She passed out in the Himalayas. Our colleague, who has suffered from sleep apnea for years, offered to share his oxygen tanks with her.

When confronted with obvious symptoms such as oxygen deficiencies and skeletal irregularities, many healthcare professionals fail to diagnose correctly. Our medical system frequently overlooks airway issues despite their prevalence and devastating fallout if left untreated. Ron Harper, a neurologist at UCLA, says simple tests could indicate problems with gray matter and prefrontal lobe function, yet they remain largely unused.

One test that dentists can use is CBCT, which is a specialized x-ray technique that provides a three-dimensional view of the craniofacial structures, including the dental arches, jawbones, and the airway. Unlike traditional two-dimensional x-rays, CBCT scans offer a more comprehensive understanding of the size, shape, and patency (openness) of the airway.

These measurements can be critical for diagnosis and be

invaluable for interdisciplinary treatments involving ortho-dontists, surgeons, and sleep specialists.

CBCT scans offer a proactive approach to airway health, helping healthcare providers and patients make informed decisions that can have lifelong benefits.

Remember, your child's journey from five to ten is about more than just growing up—it's about setting the ground-work for a lifetime of health. Understanding the signs and making informed choices can empower you to protect and prioritize your child's airway well-being.

SIX
AIRWAY HEALTH IN TEENS

Have You Noticed Your Teen Struggling to Focus or Seemingly Overwhelmed?

The teenage years are a whirlwind of emotions, changes, and challenges. Amidst all the drama and discovery, could your teenager be silently struggling with an airway health disorder? Here's a checklist to help you get to the heart of the matter:

- Is your teen still snoring, or has it gotten worse?
- Does your teen complain of persistent fatigue, even after a full night's sleep?
- Has your teen been newly diagnosed with anxiety or depression?
- Have you noticed bruxism?
- Does your teen have a scalloped tongue?
- Is there a noticeable decline in academic performance or focus?
- Do you observe frequent nighttime waking or sleep disruptions?

- Has your teen's appetite changed, especially for sugary or high-carb foods?
- Are there any symptoms of TMJ, (temporomandibular joint disorder) like jaw pain or clicking?
- Does your teen struggle with allergies, recurrent sinus infections, or respiratory issues?
- Have you noticed posture changes like hunched shoulders or forward head posture?
- Is your teen experiencing social withdrawal or decreased interest in activities they once enjoyed?

If any of these signs resonate with your teen's experience, it's crucial to consult a healthcare provider skilled in diagnosing and treating airway health disorders. In the turbulent tide of adolescence, every breath should empower them to face life's challenges, not add to them.

Teen years are often described as a rollercoaster, replete with emotional highs and lows. But what if those mood swings and an apparent lack of focus aren't just "teenage angst"? What if they're signs of an underlying airway issue that's affecting both their cognitive and emotional well-being?

Teenagers are at a crucial juncture where lifestyle habits and health interventions set the foundation for their adulthood. Understanding airway health at this stage can influence not just their immediate wellness but also their lifelong health trajectory.

Savvy's lung issues started affecting her daily routine as she entered fifth and sixth grade. Her teachers noticed her drifting away, blanking out, and requiring constant redirection. Savvy needed a strong coffee to get prepared and organized for the day. She began forgetting completed assignments in her locker and was chided by her teachers for it. Teachers scolded her for forgetting a red pen, suggesting that such forgetfulness could jeopardize her chances of college graduation.

Savvy was losing her ability to recall, a direct result of hypoxia's impact on her brain's gray matter. Instead of understanding the root cause or seeing it as a cause of concern, her sixth-grade homeroom teacher labeled her as lazy. This treatment was a stark contrast to her early school years, where she was considered one of the brightest kids, and it was difficult for Savvy to process this seemingly big change in her identity.

How many times do you take your child to the doctor and they ask how your child is sleeping? Unless you have a doctor who is well-versed in airway health, that isn't usually one of the first questions they ask. However, chronic sleep deprivation associated with airway disorders can impact cognitive development, leading to learning difficulties and behavioral problems. Imagine a world where a child's academic struggles are not dismissed as laziness or lack of effort but are instead investigated as potential signs of an underlying health issue. This change in perspective, paired with empathy and the subsequent early intervention, could dramatically alter a child's academic and personal growth trajectory.

Dr. Kotagal says that when you measure what has happened to a child's brain, especially in those first three years or thereafter with additional hypoxia, much of the issue is the ability to recall. Memory problems. They test these kids by giving them five or seven words in a row and asking them to repeat once they hear each word. If you don't have hypoxic brain dysfunction, you have no problem repeating those words. If you do have this problem, you can maybe repeat two or three words max.

Savvy once came to me stating, "Mom, I'm not smart anymore." This was devastating to hear. It was also around this time that her school performance began to decline. She had trouble remembering things, couldn't focus, and struggled with her academic workload.

The early teen years are a delicate period of growth as is, and as a result of these newfound struggles, Savvy's sense of self and potential quickly dwindled. She found herself unable to participate in sports as before and faced unexplained physical changes. Despite these alarming signs, no one could pinpoint the problem because she appeared fine.

It was not until Savvy was twelve years old that the severity of her condition became fully apparent. The orthognathic surgery finally came about when we decided to consult a psychologist friend in Seattle about Savvy. I also had a dental appointment with Dr. McKay, and so while there, I had him assess Savvy. Seeing her ten years after our initial meeting, he was taken back by the severity of her blocked airways. He examined Savvy and exclaimed, "Oh my gosh! I don't know how she breathes! Her airway is fifty to eighty percent blocked. You have to see Dr. Hang right away."

We reached out to Dr. Bill Hang for guidance. He suggested we first meet with Joy Moeller, a renowned myofunctional therapist based in Pacific Palisades and Beverly Hills. Joy redirected us to Patrick McKeown, a leading coach in breathing exercises. At six a.m., prior to going to school, Savvy would Skype with Patrick. She would be in a cold sweat from being unable to sleep well and had great difficulty trying to do the breathing exercises. Unfortunately, Savvy was unable to perform the exercises Patrick suggested, mainly due to her inability to breathe through her nose and barely through her mouth.

We flew out to Los Angeles to see Joy in person. Upon examination, Joy, using the Mallampati scale, found that Savvy's airway was actually eighty to one hundred percent blocked. The Mallampati score is a classification system used by medical professionals to predict the difficulty of intubation by assessing the size of the upper airway and the amount of mouth opening. The score ranges from Class I (most visible airway structures, suggesting easy intubation) to Class IV (least visible airway structures, indicating potential difficulty in intubation). That severity for Savvy meant it was too late for myofunctional therapy, too.

Since other therapies wouldn't work because of Savvy's advanced condition, it was decided that we would officially see Dr. Hang. He took images and called Dr. Larry Wolford in Dallas so she could be scheduled for immediate orthognathic surgery. Orthognathic surgery, also known as corrective jaw surgery, is a procedure that corrects conditions of the jaw and face related to structure, growth, sleep apnea, TMJ disorders, malocclusion problems owing to skeletal disharmonies, or other orthodontic problems that cannot be easily treated with braces.

Orthognathic surgery can reposition the upper jaw, lower jaw, or both to correct imbalances. The exact procedure will vary depending on the individual's specific needs. This may involve cutting and realigning the bones in the jaw and, in some cases, adding extra bone to the jaw.

Dr. Hang prepared Savvy for orthognathic surgery by wiring her jaws in accordance with Dr. Wolford's surgical plan. Since this severely limited her breathing, she was functional for only an hour or two each day.

Our insurance company, Blue Cross Blue Shield of Texas, said if she did not have sleep apnea, it would not reimburse for the surgery because it would be considered dental and cosmetic. Ten days before Savvy's surgery, we went to see Dr. Christian Guilleminault at Stanford Medical Center. She was too weak to walk and needed a wheelchair to get through the airports and around buildings. Dr. Guilleminault immediately ordered testing for multiple sclerosis (MS) and narcolepsy. He diagnosed her with obstructive sleep apnea.

Fortunately, Savvy's tests were negative for MS and narcolepsy, but it worked in her favor to have her surgery covered.

On December 15, 2015, Savvy became one of the youngest patients to undergo orthognathic surgery. Her recovery was arduous, with six days in the hospital and continuous travel back and forth from Dallas. However, Dr. Wolford, her surgeon, was incredibly kind and supportive. He believed in Savvy's strength and always encouraged her.

In a few days following surgery, Savvy could breathe through her nose for the first time in her life! She could close her mouth and sleep with her mouth closed. She no longer was grinding her teeth or waking up during the night with a dry mouth. She no longer suffered from sleep apnea.

Three weeks later, on January 6, Savvy was waiting outside her new school hours before it opened after Christmas break, ready to go in. Dr. Wolford had successfully repaired her craniofacial respiratory complex, allowing her to breathe normally and walk a mile to her school. She was so excited to feel normal that the principal had to break the news to her that school didn't start until the following morning. It was great to see her so excited about life again!

Consider this: from ages eight to thirteen, Savvy was unable to walk farther than a couple of short city blocks. She struggled with stairs. At our home, she resorted to moving up step by step seated on her backside. Following surgery, she could keep pace with her friends and could even walk to the nearby high school after school if she desired. Life had taken on a fresh hue for her. She still needed to rest more frequently for a while, but her stamina was gradually returning. She no longer struggled as much with memory recall. Since she was ahead of her peers due to her AP course load, she kept busy helping correct papers and tutoring classmates.

Then came a letter from President Obama, praising her for

her exceptional academic achievements. She was even nomi-
nated for the Dell UT summer pre-med program, but she
boldly told them she couldn't partake if they didn't prioritize
accurate diagnostics. Her logic was simple: if a diagnosis isn't
correct, the subsequent treatment is meaningless. She had
firsthand experience of this and knew how important it was.

At the end of eighth grade, Savvy requested a move back
to Seattle, where the air was cooler and more humid, which
she found easier to breathe. She applied to several prestigious
schools and expressed a desire for greater intellectual challenges. She felt her current environment was lacking, and she
yearned to be pushed. Eventually, she was accepted into the
Seattle Academy of Arts and Sciences on Capitol Hill.

However, once there, she had difficulty walking the steep
hills at school because the muscles needed were never really
developed. Her improved stamina wasn't able to keep up
with that kind of hilly trek.

Savvy would call me and say, "I don't know what's
wrong. I just walked up the hill for Spanish class, and my
heart is beating out of my chest. I'm scared." Other calls then
ensued, like "I can't join the volleyball team because I can't
get through fifteen minutes of the workout prep." It was as if
her body was shutting down yet again, and it was terrifying.

She tried to work through it and made efforts to adapt,
with teachers making accommodations where they could.
However, she faced difficulties, like being expected to climb
stairs to her fifth-floor science class, despite her requesting to
use the elevator, which was denied since students weren't
allowed to use it. The teachers didn't see a crutch or a wheelchair. Savvy looked fine on the outside, so her invisible
disabilities were continually misunderstood and underes-
timated.

A major turning point came when she met her new pediatrician in Seattle, Dr. Rebecca Cronin. Although trained in

Boston and specializing in adolescent girls, Dr. Cronin admitted she was unsure how to manage Savvy's complex conditions. Not yet recognizing her hypoxic brain dysfunction or connective tissue disorder, Dr. Cronin recognized that she couldn't run the tests on Savvy needed for next steps because of her age and insurance limitations. Instead, she referred us to a naturopath, Dr. Shannon Estrada, stating that she's one of the best of the best and could do the tests needed.

Dr. Estrada ran a series of tests that revealed Savvy had incredibly low levels of iron, serotonin, and other crucial brain chemicals. She also had a severe deficiency in vitamin D and DHA. Based on these findings, we immediately began treatment, including B12 injections, ten thousand units of Vitamin D daily, and various supplements. These were necessary due to Savvy's limited diet of soft foods, a result of her misaligned teeth and swallowing difficulties. This is something that a lot of kids could use, but doctors don't recognize how kids are impacted through today's diet and craniofacial structures.

Since Savvy scored high enough on her SAT at the age of twelve, when she turned sixteen, she declared she wanted to go to college. She was accepted at a top fifty private college in Walla Walla, Washington, known as Whitman College.

As winter came and there was ice and snow covering the sidewalks at Whitman, she began falling. The cold caused her joints to regularly ache, and her temporomandibular joints caused pain as well, which we attributed to her recent jaw surgery, not knowing anything more than what we were told. She was granted medical leave from Whitman College.

Dr. Wolford recommended a replacement of her temporomandibular joints, which would involve a wait of five months just to order customized titanium joints. Meanwhile, Savvy's health declined further; she ached more and more, and she grew despondent. We decided to move back to Austin to get out of the cold since it made Savvy struggle more, and the surgery would be in Dallas with Dr. Wolford anyhow.

After the TMJ surgery and feeling slightly better, in September 2019, despite already attending college, Savvy chose to attend McCallum High School to have the full and normal experience of a senior year among her old friends. On one of the first days, she was forced to rush to the bathroom, vomiting loudly within earshot of her classmates. It was embarrassing for her when all she wanted was to feel like she fit in. This incident, along with her constant sickness that arose once she started attending the school, led us to seek help from Dr. Becky Andrews, a naturopathic practitioner.

Dr. Becky immediately suspected that Savvy had Hypermobile Ehlers-Danlos syndrome (hEDS) based on certain physical characteristics from her eyes to her knees to her ankles. To our surprise, Dr. Becky also noticed that she exhibited signs of Adderall addiction. While Savvy was at Whitman College, she was introduced to it by a friend and found it helped her concentrate. Dr. Becky likened the effects of Adderall on Savvy's brain to pouring crack cocaine on it.

Around the same time, Dr. Becky identified that McCallum High School, like many others in Austin, was riddled with mold—a potential trigger for Savvy's mast cell activation syndrome (MCAS). Many of the schools are built with flat roofs, which was the style in the 1950s and 1960s when they were built. When it rains, water can seep down the inside walls of the school, and if you walk through the halls, you may see black fuzz on the ceiling tiles. We soon learned that mold is known to exacerbate symptoms in hEDS patients, making the environment at the school hazardous for Savvy.

Needless to say, this was a disappointing discovery since we had just moved there so Savvy could have the best senior year possible by being reunited with her old friends. It was disheartening to see her struggle after all she had been through, including her TMJ replacement surgery and subsequent recovery.

A few years later, I asked Dr. Hang why Savvy still had issues with concentration, memory, panic attacks, and physical stamina despite the corrective actions. He said, "It is kind of like a wildfire. It starts with smoke—when a child isn't breathing and sleeping well—and roars into a fire the longer it is before their airway is corrected." Dr. Kotagal once said, "It's so sad that teenagers who have suffered for years from a compromised airway and sleep apnea can be the most difficult to help."

There comes a point when we can't afford to put off our child's health concerns, no matter what. Most of us realize when there is a deeper problem arising with our kids, and we know it's not normal, even when everyone else may be saying it is. You have to follow your gut and keep pushing because the experts we surround ourselves with may not be the experts in what your child actually needs help with.

There is also a proven link between airway disorders and ADHD (attention deficit hyperactivity disorder). ADHD has been viewed primarily through the lens of neurobiology and psychology. Symptoms such as inattention, hyperactivity, and impulsivity are the main focus of diagnosis and subsequent treatment, usually involving behavioral therapy and medication like stimulants. However, emerging research suggests that airway issues like sleep apnea, mouth breathing, and other forms of sleep-disordered breathing may contribute to or exacerbate ADHD symptoms.

Why might this be the case? Poor airway health can lead to fragmented, low-quality sleep. When children or adults don't get restorative sleep, they can experience a range of cognitive and behavioral issues that closely mimic the symptoms of ADHD, such as difficulty concentrating, impulsivity, and hyperactivity. Moreover, inadequate oxygen intake—known as hypoxia—can affect brain function and development, which could contribute to neurological symptoms.

Studies indicate that some children diagnosed with ADHD show significant improvement in their symptoms after undergoing treatment for airway issues. This treatment often involves the use of continuous positive airway pressure (CPAP) devices, orthodontic intervention, or even surgical removal of the adenoids and tonsils to improve airway flow.

Moreover, clinicians are starting to pay more attention to symptoms that overlap between airway issues and ADHD, such as daytime sleepiness, irritability, and trouble focusing. Some experts advocate for sleep studies or airway assessments as part of the diagnostic process for ADHD.

The potential connection between airway health and ADHD opens up a new frontier in holistic healthcare. It suggests that for some individuals, addressing airway issues could be a critical component in managing ADHD symptoms, possibly reducing the need for medication.

If your teenager has struggled with airway disorders for years and you haven't recognized it, I don't want you to feel like it's too late. Getting them assessed by an airway health professional is the most important step to take, and then you can determine what the next best steps may be. For some teens, surgery may be the most effective intervention for significant airway issues. However, non-invasive methods like continued jaw and palate expansion and myofunctional therapy should be seriously considered before opting for surgical routes.

The teen years are complex, but they also offer a vital window for intervention that can set the stage for a healthier, happier adult life. This chapter may not be the easiest to navigate, but it could be one of the most important in your teen's life story.

DR. LARRY WOLFORD - MESSAGE TO THE READER
AIRWAY OBSTRUCTION

By Dr. Larry Wolford, DMD,
Leading Oral and Maxillofacial Surgeon

ORAL AND MAXILLOFACIAL SURGERY PERSPECTIVE

Airway obstruction at birth can lead to devastating outcomes such as brain injury, neuromuscular disorders, failure to thrive, and death. The obstetric delivery team needs to be prepared to manage these initial airway emergencies. A universal airway screening protocol must be developed and applied for every newborn, as early detection of obstruction and intervention will provide the best outcome for each infant. A pre-delivery ultrasound to evaluate the facial morphology may alert the delivery team of a potential airway crisis for better preparation of airway management at birth. Airway obstruction can occur in the upper airway (nose, mouth, and oropharyngeal area) or lower airway from the trachea to the lungs. The upper airway will be the focus of this document.

Upper airway obstruction can be present at birth or

develop in childhood, teenage years, or adulthood. Newborns with a recessed mandible (lower jaw) are particularly susceptible to airway difficulties. However, normal-appearing babies may have hidden obstructions related to enlargement of the tonsils, adenoid tissues, tongue, and/or soft palate/uvula, or rarely tumors in the airway. Congenital deformities causing obstructive sleep apnea at birth include hundreds of syndromes, with the more common being hemifacial microsomia, Treacher Collins syndrome, Pierre Robin anomaly, Nager syndrome, Crouzon and Apert syndromes, etc. These conditions can cause severe restriction of the oropharyngeal and nasal airways that can cause significant hypoxia (lack of oxygen) with potentially devastating consequences if not identified immediately and appropriately managed. Newborns with airway issues need prompt securing of the airway and may require endotracheal intubation or tracheostomy for survival until other appropriate interventions can be applied. Advances in distraction technology of the upper and lower jaws may be helpful in the early stages of these patients to increase the oropharyngeal airway.

Some airway issues outside of the syndrome group that can develop in childhood and teenage years would include genetic factors with small retruded jaws; trauma, particularly fractures of the mandibular condylar process with immediate recession of the mandible; growth inhibition conditions; TMJ ankylosis (frozen jaws); and TMJ pathologies that cause mandibular condylar resorption, resulting in progressive recession of the mandible. Any of these conditions can increase the risk of obstructive sleep apnea (OSA).

The upper airway areas of potential obstruction will be addressed systematically, beginning with the nose, oral cavity, and oropharyngeal structures. Partial or complete blockage in one or more of these anatomical regions can contribute to

OSA and in infancy, childhood, and teenage years can result in facial deformity, brain damage, learning disabilities, neuro-muscular disorders, and death.

NASAL AIRWAY OBSTRUCTION

Common abnormal anatomical structures that can contribute to nasal obstruction include: 1) Hyperplastic infe-rior turbinates; 2) Deviated nasal septum; 3) Narrow width of nostrils; 4) Collapse of the lateral nasal cartilages (nasal valves); and 5) Nasal polyps. Nasal airway obstruction in childhood and early teens can adversely affect the growth and development of the facial structures resulting in: 1) Vertical lengthening of the face; 2) Recessed mandible and maxilla; 3) Narrow dental arches; 4) Anterior open bite; 5) Difficulty to close lips (lip incompetence); 6) Posterior displacement of the tongue; 7) Obligate mouth breathing, and 8) Decreased oropharyngeal airway and OSA.

The indicated surgical procedures to address the nasal airway obstruction include: 1) Partial reduction of the nasal inferior turbinates; 2) Nasoseptoplasty; 3) Columella recon-struction; 4) Nasal valves reconstruction; and 5) Remove nasal polyps.

ORAL CAVITY CONTRIBUTORY FACTORS TO OSA

Oral cavity anatomical variations contributing to OSA may decrease available oral cavity volume to accommodate the tongue, subsequently displacing it posteriorly into the oropharyngeal space, impeding airway flow. Contributory factors may include: 1) retruded mandible and maxilla; 2) transverse constriction on the dental arches; 3) macroglossia (large tongue); 4) mandibular tori and palatal torus (abnormal bone growths diminishing the oral cavity space); 5) tongue-tie; and 6) unnecessary orthodontic extraction of bicuspid teeth.

Indicated procedures to address these issues include: 1) orthognathic surgery to advance the mandible and maxilla (predictably opens the oropharyngeal airway); 2) orthodontic treatment to expand the upper and lower arches, sometimes augmented with adjunctive surgical procedures to facilitate the expansion; 3) reduction glossectomy (tongue size reduction); 4) removal of mandibular tori and maxillary torus; 5) release and repair of the tongue-tie; and 6) avoid unnecessary dental extractions.

EFFECTS OF ORTHODONTICS ON THE AIRWAY

A common fallacy in orthodontics occurs when the maxilla is in a relatively normal position, but the mandible is recessed. Instead of orthognathic surgery to advance the mandible, some orthodontists will extract bicuspid teeth and retract the maxillary teeth to align with the recessed mandibular teeth, significantly reducing the oral cavity volume and displacing the tongue into the oropharyngeal space, decreasing the airway. For some patients, this treatment will induce sleep apnea with a major negative impact on the patients breathing, health, well-being, and facial balance. Although there are necessary indications where permanent teeth need to be extracted in order to align the remaining teeth, bicuspid extraction should be avoided in teenagers and adults, particularly if the jaws are recessed.

OROPHARYNGEAL OBSTRUCTION

The common anatomical factors contributory to a decrease in the oropharyngeal airway space that can produce OSA include: 1) recessed mandible and maxilla displacing the tongue into the oropharyngeal space; 2) macroglossia; 3) hyperplastic tonsils; 4) hyperplastic adenoid tissue; 5) hyperplastic soft palate/uvula; and 6) tumors.

Indicated procedures to address these anatomical variations include: 1) mandibular and maxillary osteotomies for advancement (highly predictable to increase the oropharyngeal airway; 2) partial glossectomy (reduction of tongue size); 3) tonsillectomy; 4) adenoidectomy; 5) uvulopalatopharyngoplasty (UPPP) to reduce soft palate/uvula size; and 6) tumor removal.

In young children with sleep apnea, tonsillectomy and adenoidectomy may be indicated early in life to improve the airway. Hyperplastic turbinates are very common in patients with OSA, and reduction may also be indicated in childhood, adolescence or adulthood to improve the nasal airway. Nasal airway obstruction can cause habitual mouth breathing with a profound effect on a child's facial growth and development. Identifying the nasal airway and oropharyngeal obstructions may be indicated for early treatment to improve nasal airway function, decreasing the adverse effect on facial growth and development. However, performing nasoseptoplasty prior to the mid-teenage years could have an adverse effect on maxillary growth.

THE ROLE OF THE TMJs (JAW JOINTS) IN AIRWAY OBSTRUCTION

The temporomandibular joints (TMJs) are the foundation for: 1) jaw position and occlusal stability; 2) facial balance; 3) jaw and jaw joint function; 4) facial growth and development; 5) airway function; 6) maintain comfort without associated pain factors; and 7) stability for orthodontic and orthognathic surgery outcomes. TMJ abnormality or pathology can adversely affect any or all of these factors.

In relation to sleep apnea, conditions affecting jaw position and the airway may involve genetics resulting in underdevelopment of the mandible and/or TMJ pathology that can cause a normal mandible to become progressively receded with resorption of the mandibular condyles, creating significant facial deformity and airway compromise. These conditions include:

1. Juvenile idiopathic arthritis (JIA) occurs more commonly in females, with onset in early childhood to age sixteen years old and is a connective tissue autoimmune disease.

2. Adolescent internal condylar resorption (AICR) affects predominantly females with onset during pubertal growth.

3. Reactive arthritis, a low-grade infection in the TMJ caused by bacteria and viruses. It can affect teenagers and adults.

4. Trauma to the mandible with fractures of the condyles resulting in immediate recession of the mandible with adverse effects on function and mandibular growth.

5. Ankylosis (fusion of the upper and lower jaw at the TMJ) when occurring early in life can result in severe underdevelopment of the mandible affecting the airway as well as significant difficulties with jaw function, oral hygiene, and nutrition.

6. Other connective autoimmune diseases that can cause condylar resorption include psoriatic arthritis, rheumatoid arthritis, scleroderma, lupus, Sjogren's syndrome, etc. Some of these conditions occur more commonly in adults but can occur in the teenage years or younger.

For newborns with major airway obstruction, securing the airway with endotracheal intubation or a tracheostomy may be necessary initially for airway management and survival. Subsequently, distraction osteogenesis could be employed to lengthen the mandible and improve the airway, but this is not without potential risks. Young patients and those in the adolescent years that sustain fractures of the mandibular condyles will have the best outcome for mandibular function, growth, and airway stability by having the condylar fractures surgically reduced and stabilized. Condylar fractures left unattended can result in immediate jaw retrusion, decreased oropharyngeal airway, and potential interference of facial growth.

Patients with healthy TMJs and sleep apnea related to retruded mandible and maxilla can benefit from surgery to advance the jaws forward in a counterclockwise direction. This increases the oropharyngeal airway dimensions and is the most predictable method to eliminate OSA for many patients. Patients who have had previously untreated mandibular condylar fractures, advanced TMJ pathology such as in AICR, reactive arthritis, ankylosis, connective tissue autoimmune diseases, etc., the most predictable treatment to advance the mandible forward with or counterclockwise rotation is the application of custom TMJ total joint prostheses (Stryker TMJ Concepts, Inc., Ventura CA) in conjunction with maxilla surgery. This author has used these devices for over 34 years and has not had to replace any for wear or failure. The devices may have the potential to last a lifetime. For end-stage TMJ conditions, total joint prostheses are the only method to create good stability and function, eliminating associated pain and sleep apnea.

CONCLUSIONS

Airway obstruction at birth can lead to devastating outcomes such as brain injury, neuromuscular disorders, failure to thrive, and death. A universal airway screening process must be developed and applied for every newborn because recognizing obstruction and early intervention will provide the best outcome for each baby. The goals in managing obstructive sleep apnea are to identify it in the newborn when present with quick, decisive action for airway control. This should mitigate irreversible consequences of hypoxia. OSA can also develop during childhood and in the teen years, and in adults associated with recessed jaws commonly associated with condylar resorption. Contributory factors for OSA are often multifactorial and must be identified with appropriate development of a treatment protocol to address the involved factors. TMJ pathology developing in childhood, teenage years, or as an adult related to condylar resorption can create major dentofacial deformities and OSA. TMJ reconstruction and mandibular advancement with custom TMJ total joint prostheses in conjunction with maxillary surgery can restore facial balance, improve jaw function, and eliminate pain as well as OSA.

SEVEN

THE COMPOUNDING IMPACT OF AIRWAY DISORDERS

With Savvy's condition worsening yet again so severely, she was on the verge of giving up. Desperate for guidance, I reached out to Joy Moeller again. She suggested we consult directly with Dr. Suresh Kotagal, since he specializes in sleep medicine and airway issues at Mayo Clinic in Rochester. Dr. Kotagal had been directly educated by Dr. Gulliemineau, who is considered the father of sleep apnea. I was overwhelmed with excitement and hoped for a cure because, being a proud Minnesotan, I consider Mayo Clinic Rochester the best in the world. I immediately arranged for a visit.

During February 2019 at Mayo Clinic Rochester, Dr. Kotagal wasted no time in diagnosing Savvy with an autonomic disorder. This was a breakthrough, as it shed light on the connection between airway issues and autonomic dysfunction—an area rarely discussed. A tilt table test that shot her heart rate up to one hundred and sixty beats per minute confirmed Savvy's diagnosis of postural orthostatic tachycardia syndrome (POTS). He also diagnosed her with restless leg syndrome and an iron deficiency. Following brain and spinal MRIs, she was referred to a rheumatologist, Dr.

Amir Orandi, who suspected a patellofemoral disorder due to symptoms in her feet and knees, which was later confirmed. Once all the images were gathered, Savvy was sent to a Mayo psychologist who could show her what was going on in her body and brain, as well as why she was experiencing anxiety, depression, and medical PTSD. This was a breakthrough. Talking with someone who actually understood her chronic health issues and the toll they were taking on her physical and mental health was validating and profoundly helpful.

A year later, we visited Texas Children's again, which led to the official diagnoses of hEDS from Dr. Brendan Lee, a renowned geneticist and chair of the largest genetics and genomics lab in the nation, which operates at both Baylor College of Medicine in Houston and Texas Children's. Dr. Lee's expertise in rare diseases made him a valuable resource, as he had knowledge of rare disorders that few others possessed.

The diagnostic process involved various physical tests, such as assessing Savvy's flexibility and joint mobility. These evaluations checked if she could touch her palms to the floor while bending over and if she could pull her thumb all the way down to her wrist. A score of five or more on these tests, along with her narrative, indicated a diagnosis of hEDS. Genetic testing further supplemented the diagnosis.

The average time for hEDS diagnosis had decreased from sixteen to twelve years. Once thought to impact every one in 500,000 people, it has been revised to one in 5,000.[1]

On February 14, 2020, Valentine's Day, we received Savvy's diagnosis amidst the emerging fear and uncertainty surrounding the COVID-19 pandemic. As much as knowing specifically what was happening with her was a relief, it also was filled with great sadness. The hEDS diagnosis was associated with the potential need for mobility aids such as wheelchairs, crutches, or canes; chronic pain and frequent joint dislocations were common symptoms for life. She was too young to have to endure all of this. Depression loomed over Savvy after she got her diagnosis of hEDS.

One afternoon, Savvy's shoulder dislocated, prompting me to rush to a nearby Walgreens to fetch a sling, walker, transfer chair, knee braces, ankle braces, and other necessary supplies. A few days later, a nurse caseworker from United-Healthcare advised me to never show my sadness about the situation, so I put on a brave face and focused on finding solutions. Savvy soon learned to relocate her own shoulder, a skill she honed over time.

It is critical to understand that airway disorders in children, while primarily manifesting as physical symptoms, can also deeply impact a child's mental health. Over time, these physical health issues can lead to significant psychological distress and even mental health disorders such as depression.

Research indicates that children with airway disorders often exhibit a higher prevalence of mental health issues compared to their peers without these disorders.[2] The chronic nature of airway disorders can disrupt a child's daily life in multiple ways, which, over time, contribute to feelings of sadness, hopelessness, and other depressive symptoms.

One of the main factors at play here is the disruption of normal physiological processes. For example, OSA can affect oxygen saturation levels and disrupt neurotransmitter regulation in the brain. Sleep deprivation can interfere with the neurochemical processes that regulate emotions, increasing the likelihood of depressive symptoms in children.

The significance of sleep disorders cannot be overstated. After reading *Why We Sleep* by Matthew Walker, I realized that Savvy's condition aligned with the stories shared in the book. Sleep disorders contribute to various issues like ADD, ADHD, substance abuse, and even suicidality. The consequences of untreated sleep and airway disorders on long-term health are alarming.

Beyond the physical challenges, the psychological burden of dealing with an airway disorder can be profound. Children might feel different from their peers or face limitations in physical activities, which can lead to negative self-perception, lower self-esteem, and overall psychological distress. These experiences may further increase the risk of depression.

Discussing topics such as suicide, substance abuse, and similar sensitive issues is vital, as it resonates deeply with many individuals. This point is clearly supported in Dr. Kotagal's research, which reveals that certain populations are more likely to experience specific issues, like a four percent increased likelihood of engaging in substance abuse or a fifteen percent increased probability of living with chronic pain. The surrounding people may not fully comprehend the severity of their pain, leaving them feeling isolated and misunderstood.

Consider Savvy, for instance. After having her retractive orthodontics and palate expander removed at the age of nine, her health took a turn for the worse. She could barely walk a short city block without getting winded, she struggled to climb stairs, she started forgetting her homework, and generally her world began to crumble. Just a year before, she was an energetic child running up hills in Florence, Italy. Now she was grouped with children suffering from severe conditions like leukemia. She felt unintelligent; her body was failing her, and she didn't understand what was happening.

As a parent, I want to emphasize that not only do we, as parents, struggle to comprehend the gravity of our children's conditions, but even the medical professionals often fail to understand. Dr. Andrew Maxwell, a pediatric cardiologist and hEDS specialist, highlights the unfortunate reality faced by children like Savvy. They undergo immense medical abuse, being told that their multitude of symptoms is an exaggeration or that they are mentally unstable. It's disheartening to witness the lack of empathy and understanding from many healthcare professionals.

Should your child exhibit depressive symptoms, there are several therapeutic interventions available, including cognitive behavioral therapy (CBT), play therapy, and family therapy. These approaches aim to manage emotional difficulties, bolster coping strategies, and encourage resilience within children and their families.

Given these complex interactions, it's crucial that routine mental health screenings are integrated into the overall evaluation and treatment plan for children with airway disorders. By using validated screening tools and thorough clinical assessments, healthcare professionals can better identify children who may be at risk of developing depressive symptoms or already experiencing them.

EIGHT
SYSTEMIC HEALTH AND MULTIDISCIPLINARY TEAMS

In 2022, walking into the bustling room of a major national medical and dental conference, I was greeted by a sea of faces, all engrossed in discussions surrounding the mouth and the craniofacial respiratory complex. However, what struck me was the glaring absence of any dialogue about systemic disorders arising from children's airway and sleep issues.

Some of these professionals seemed oblivious to the hypoxic injuries that can lead to dysautonomia, connective tissue disorders, muscular degeneration, or stunted growth of cartilage and muscles due to inadequate oxygenation. I couldn't help but wonder how many correct diagnoses are being missed as a result because I know firsthand how devastating those misdiagnoses can be.

Savvy was slowly suffering right in front of my eyes for years. Hypoxic injuries occurred to her body and brain from the airway disorders, and her endothelial system was unable to deliver sufficient oxygen to her muscles. Compounded with a collagen issue, her thinning tissue, musculature, and ligaments could not properly support her joints. Consequently, this affected her feet, knees, hips, and overall growth.

Dr. Suresh Kotagal, a leading pediatric neurologist at Mayo Rochester who has been involved in Savvy's care since 2019, is of the firm belief that the systemic damage caused by hypoxic dysfunction can lead to crippling disorders. He was the first to diagnose Savvy with POTS and argued that her condition was not limited to craniofacial-respiratory issues but was systemic, a fact that even the medical professionals aware of the dire impact of airway dysfunctions do not seem to agree on.

Sadly, the diagnosis and treatment of the craniofacial respiratory complex often overshadows the underlying damage caused to the brain and body due to hypoxic injuries. The resulting brain damage is most worrying, given the irreversible nature of its effects on a child's intellectual capabilities. Savvy, despite her exceptionally high IQ, began to struggle academically. For many children who aren't constantly breathing and sleeping properly as they grow, the loss of IQ points can be devastating.

The connection between conditions like idiopathic condylar resorption and hEDS with airway health offers a window into the intricate relationship between oral health and systemic well-being. When the structures of the mouth and jaw are affected, as they are in idiopathic condylar resorption, it's not merely a localized issue. Such imbalances can disrupt breathing, potentially leading to sleep apnea or other airway disorders, and thereby contribute to neurocognitive issues like ADHD. These physiological changes can, in turn, impact the brain's function, exacerbating symptoms of conditions related to cognitive and systemic development.

The interconnectedness of the mouth and overall health gives credence to the idea that imbalances in one area can ripple through various physiological systems. For example, poor oral posture or breathing difficulties can lead to imbalances in the autonomic nervous system, affecting how the body manages stress, inflammation, and other critical functions. In this way, oral health serves as a sort of bellwether for broader health issues.

Understanding these interconnections is crucial for healthcare professionals as they devise more holistic treatment plans. It suggests the need for cross-disciplinary approaches that address not just the symptomatic manifestations of conditions like ADHD or hEDS but also underlying issues that may contribute to them. As research continues, the medical community is likely to uncover even more links between oral health and systemic conditions, illuminating new pathways for effective treatment and early intervention.

The American Academy of Oral Systemic Health (AAOSH) also stresses that such conditions are systemic, not isolated.[1] Let's break down the systemic effects:

- **Cardiovascular System:** Children with airway disorders, such as OSA, often experience recurrent episodes of partial or complete airway obstruction during sleep. These episodes can lead to intermittent hypoxia, increased carbon dioxide levels, and fluctuations in intrathoracic pressure. Over time, these physiological disturbances can contribute to cardiovascular complications, including systemic hypertension, endothelial dysfunction, and increased risk of cardiovascular disease later in life.

- **Cardiac Function:** The intermittent oxygen desaturation and elevated carbon dioxide levels associated with airway disorders can strain the cardiovascular system, leading to increased workload on the heart. This increased workload may result in cardiac remodeling, impaired ventricular function, and an increased risk of arrhythmia in children with airway disorders.

- **Neurocognitive Function:** Children with airway disorders often experience disrupted sleep patterns, including frequent awakenings, sleep fragmentation, and decreased total sleep time. The resulting sleep deprivation and poor sleep quality can lead to cognitive impairments, including deficits in attention, memory, executive functioning, and academic performance. Early intervention and effective management of airway disorders are crucial for optimizing neurocognitive development in these children.[2]

- **Behavioral and Emotional Impact:** Sleep disruption caused by airway disorders can also contribute to behavioral and emotional difficulties in children. Increased irritability, mood swings, hyperactivity, and ADHD-like symptoms are commonly observed. Addressing and treating airway disorders can significantly improve behavioral and emotional well-being in affected children.

- **Growth and Development:** Airway disorders, especially when associated with feeding difficulties or chronic mouth breathing, can impact a child's nutritional status and growth. Inadequate oxygenation, decreased appetite, and energy expenditure during respiratory efforts can contribute to growth retardation and delayed physical development. Timely intervention, nutritional support, and addressing airway abnormalities are crucial to promoting healthy growth in children with airway disorders.

- **Facial and Dental Development:** Chronic mouth breathing, often observed in children with airway disorders, can lead to changes in facial growth and dental alignment. The altered resting posture of the tongue, reduced nasal breathing, and increased pressure on the developing oral structures can result in narrow dental arches, malocclusions, and facial abnormalities. Early diagnosis and appropriate management of airway disorders can help mitigate these effects and support proper facial and dental development.

The lack of recognition and knowledge of these connections is what makes this situation challenging. Parents should be vigilant, even when it seems everything is developing correctly. It's important to remember that these conditions can lie dormant. This vigilance includes awareness about tooth extractions and retractable orthodontics, which can shrink the oral cavity, leaving less room for the tongue, which in turn can further block the airway and lead to a lifetime of sleep apnea.

It's not widely understood how interconnected our bodies are and how a small issue can have large-scale effects. Savvy herself, despite displaying concerning symptoms, was repeatedly reassured that everything was normal and that she would grow out of it.

Recognizing the interconnectedness between the respiratory system and various physiological systems is crucial in providing comprehensive care for children with airway disorders. Timely intervention and multidisciplinary collaboration will make the biggest difference.

When facing airway health disorders in children, the value of a cohesive, multidisciplinary approach cannot be overstated. Much like an orchestra where each instrument plays a unique role in creating a harmonious symphony, every healthcare professional in a multidisciplinary team contributes their unique expertise to help manage and improve a child's airway health.

- At the forefront, pediatricians are typically the first point of contact, as they are often the ones to do annual checks, which is why it's so important that they spot the early signs of potential airway disorders during regular check-ups. They play a pivotal role in early detection, management of symptoms, and initiating referrals to specialists as needed.

- A pediatric pulmonologist who specializes in respiratory issues can further diagnose and treat specific airway disorders. They can provide treatments such as inhalers or nebulizers and guide parents on breathing exercises and lifestyle modifications that can help improve a child's respiratory health.

- Allergists can identify and manage allergies that may contribute to or exacerbate airway disorders. They are integral in providing treatments such as antihistamines, nasal steroids, or even immunotherapy, aiming to minimize the impact of allergens on the child's airway.

- Ear, nose, and throat (ENT) specialists can address structural issues in the airway that may be causing or contributing to the problem. In certain cases, surgical intervention may be necessary to alleviate symptoms and improve airflow.

- Speech-language pathologists (SLPs) have an important role too. They can help manage swallowing disorders that might arise from or contribute to airway disorders and can also guide children and parents on exercises to strengthen oral muscles and improve swallowing and breathing.

- Dentists, particularly those specializing in airway health or pediatric dentistry are experts in airway-centric orthodontics, can assess and manage oral and dental conditions that may affect airway health. This may involve treatments to correct misaligned teeth or jaws or the use of oral appliances to maintain an open and unobstructed airway.

- Sleep specialists are also a vital part of the team. They can identify and manage sleep disorders that often go hand in hand with airway issues, ensuring that a child gets quality, restful sleep.

- Myofunctional therapists play a pivotal role in addressing the functional issues that affect the oral and facial muscles. These professionals teach children exercises to improve the strength and coordination of the muscles involved in breathing, swallowing, and articulating speech. This helps alleviate symptoms of airway disorders and improve overall airway function.

- Nutritionists or dietitians are important as they provide guidance on dietary changes that can reduce inflammation and mucus production, both of which exacerbate airway disorders. They can also offer advice on maintaining a healthy weight, as obesity is a known risk factor for many airway disorders.

- Physical therapists can help improve overall body posture and chest wall mobility, factors that significantly affect breathing and airway function. They can guide patients through exercises that strengthen respiratory muscles and improve breathing mechanics.

- Psychologists or mental health counselors may be needed to help children and families cope with the emotional and psychological challenges of dealing with a chronic airway disorder. They can provide strategies for stress management and coping with any feelings of anxiety or depression that might arise.

- Audiologists might be involved if the child has recurring ear infections, a common occurrence in children with certain airway disorders. They can assess hearing and, if necessary, arrange for the placement of ear tubes to help prevent future infections.

- Genetic counselors can provide valuable insight when there's a known or suspected genetic component to a child's airway disorder. They can guide families through the process of genetic testing and help interpret the results.

A multidisciplinary team provides a myriad of therapies and solutions, working together to ensure a child's airway health is managed effectively. By understanding the roles of each specialist, parents can actively engage in their child's care, encouraging a collaborative effort that promotes optimal health and well-being for their child.

Obtaining a detailed medical history is a crucial step in diagnosing children with obstructive breathing disorders. This includes gathering information about the child's symptoms, their duration and frequency, and any triggering factors. A comprehensive clinical evaluation, involving a thorough physical examination, focuses on assessing respiratory function, identifying signs of airway obstruction, and evaluating associated symptoms.

To confirm the presence of obstructive breathing disorders and determine their underlying causes, various diagnostic tests and tools are utilized. These include:

- **Polysomnography:** Polysomnography is considered the gold standard for diagnosing obstructive sleep apnea. It involves monitoring various physiological parameters during sleep, such as airflow, oxygen saturation, and brain activity, to evaluate the frequency and severity of respiratory events.

- **Pulmonary Function Tests (spirometry):** Spirometry measures lung function, aiding in the diagnosis of asthma and assessing the severity of airflow limitation. It measures parameters such as forced vital capacity (FVC), forced expiratory volume in one second (FEV1), and peak expiratory flow rate (PEFR).

- **Imaging Studies:** X-rays, computed tomography (CT), and magnetic resonance imaging scans (MRI) may be utilized to identify structural abnormalities in the airway, assess the extent of obstruction, and determine the appropriate management approach.

- **Sleep Studies**: Sleep studies, including home sleep apnea testing, play a crucial role in diagnosing obstructive sleep apnea in children. These studies involve monitoring sleep patterns, respiratory events, and oxygen levels during overnight sleep. The collected data, such as the apnea-hypopnea index (AHI) and oxygen saturation levels, help evaluate the severity of the condition and guide treatment decisions.

- **Mallampati Score:** The Mallampati score is a clinical tool used to predict the ease of endotracheal intubation, but it can also give indications of potential sleep apnea. It's based on the visibility of specific structures in the back of the mouth and throat when the patient opens their mouth as wide as possible and sticks out their tongue. A higher Mallampati score (class III or IV) is associated with an increased likelihood of obstructive sleep apnea.

- **Flexible Laryngoscopy:** A flexible laryngoscopy is a procedure that allows the doctor to look at the throat and larynx (voice box). It's useful for identifying structural abnormalities or issues like vocal cord dysfunction, masses, or airway obstruction.

- **Nasal Endoscopy:** This procedure enables the visualization of the nasal passages and the upper airway. It can help identify structural issues such as nasal polyps, deviated septum, or enlarged adenoids, which can contribute to airway disorders.

- **Allergy Testing:** Since allergies can contribute to airway disorders, allergy testing (skin prick or blood tests) may be used to identify specific allergens.

- **CBCT Scans:** Cone beam computed tomography (CBCT) is a type of x-ray used specifically in dentistry and orthodontics and provides a three-dimensional view of the teeth, jaw, and airway. It can be used to identify structural and anatomical factors contributing to airway disorders, such as malocclusion or narrow airways.

- **Functional Respiratory Imaging (FRI):** FRI is a novel approach combining high-resolution computed tomography (CT) imaging with computational fluid dynamics to assess the functional aspects of the respiratory system, allowing for personalized treatment strategies.

- **Body Plethysmography:** This test provides comprehensive information about the lungs and respiratory system. It's useful for diagnosing conditions like asthma and other disorders that affect lung volumes.

- **Cephalometric Analysis:** A cephalometric x-ray, often used in orthodontics, can provide valuable information about the relationship between the dental and skeletal elements of the head and neck, offering clues about potential obstructions in the airway.

Non-invasive treatment approaches aim to alleviate symptoms, improve respiratory function, and enhance the overall well-being of children with obstructive breathing disorders. These strategies may include:

- **Lifestyle Modifications:** Encouraging healthy lifestyle habits, such as weight management, regular exercise, and avoidance of triggers (e.g., allergens or pollutants), can have a positive impact on respiratory health.

- **Continuous Positive Airway Pressure (CPAP):** CPAP therapy is a treatment for moderate to severe obstructive sleep apnea. It involves wearing a mask connected to a machine that delivers pressurized air, keeping the airway open during sleep.

- **Dental and Orthodontic Interventions:** Orthodontic devices, such as palatal expanders or mandibular advancement appliances, may be recommended to help maintain an open airway.

- **Myofunctional Therapy:** This therapy involves exercises that retrain the muscles of the mouth and face. It works by improving muscle tone and reducing obstructions in the airway. They can also help with exercises to improve swallowing and breathing.

For certain cases of obstructive breathing disorders that do not respond to non-invasive treatments or present with structural abnormalities, surgical interventions may be necessary. These procedures aim to correct anatomical defects, remove obstructions, or improve airflow. Surgical options may include:

- **Airway Reconstruction**: In complex cases of congenital airway anomalies, airway reconstruction procedures may be performed to improve airway patency and alleviate breathing difficulties.

- **Turbinate Reduction**: Turbinate reduction surgery aims to reduce the size of swollen nasal turbinates, improving nasal airflow and reducing nasal congestion.

- **Tonsillectomy and Adenoidectomy**: Surgical removal of enlarged tonsils and adenoids can significantly improve airway obstruction and relieve symptoms of obstructive sleep apnea and adenotonsillar hypertrophy.

Since the challenges faced by children with airway disorders extend beyond physical symptoms, they often experience anger and frustration due to their condition. We need to also address the psychological aspects of these children's conditions. Chronic pain and systemic issues lead to heightened anxiety and depression. Ten percent of these children fall within the ten percent of Americans who struggle with depression. In many cases, these children are medicated heavily without addressing the root causes of their struggles.

When professionals from different fields share knowledge and information, they are able to facilitate a more comprehensive understanding of a child's health. It's about ensuring that every health check-up includes an assessment of the airway, every dental visit evaluates the child's breathing and sleep patterns, and every parent is aware of the signs to look for.

The challenge lies in bridging the gap between specialized multidisciplinary teams and incorporating this comprehensive approach into medical education. As we consider ways for parents to make a difference, it is crucial to learn from the textbook initiatives in Europe. Institutions like Stanford and Harvard have made significant strides in neurology and sleep medicine. By examining their successful approaches, particularly in the multidisciplinary collaboration between neurologists, DMDs, ENTs, and psychologists trained in chronic illness, we can begin to understand what makes these institutions excel. Children's hospitals should consider this approach and prioritize neurology and sleep medicine expertise to provide comprehensive care.

We know how to do this. The protocols for screening, evaluating, and treating exist and must become available to all. We must make sure that our healthcare providers, teachers, and anyone who routinely encounters our children learn to recognize and understand these infants, toddlers, and preschool children before the age of six, so they are not labeled as having behavioral problems or being lazy or stupid —they are not! We need to save them! As parents, we can learn how to recognize the symptoms, become knowledge-able advocates, and change the field of medicine and dentistry into multidisciplinary teams that give all kids a chance to become the very best they can be!

NINE
A PUBLIC HEALTH IMPERATIVE: FOCUS ON PREVENTION

"Modern medicine still does not understand the truth about the human mind and body. Doctors are trained to treat disease. And so human beings are treated like mechanical objects as doctors treat the result and not the cause."[1]

-AN EXCERPT FROM *THE 7 TOOLS OF HEALING* BY DR. STEVEN M. HALL)

Airway disorders are far more than just personal or family afflictions; they have escalated into a public health crisis that affects our communities on a grand scale. Untreated conditions like sleep apnea and chronic mouth breathing can catalyze a myriad of other health complications, from cardiovascular issues to developmental setbacks in children and even a decline in workforce productivity.

Taking action on airway health isn't just a personal endeavor—it's a societal obligation.

In 2015, Joy Moeller informed me about the first World Congress on myofunctional therapy, scheduled to take place in Los Angeles. Intrigued and wanting to learn more about Savvy's upcoming surgeries and prognosis at the time, I decided to attend. It was during this event that I met Marc Moeller, Joy's son, who organized the congress. Marc had successfully invited Dr. Christian Guilleminault to be the keynote speaker. Christian's presence attracted a wide range of professionals, including neurologists, psychiatrists, and researchers from around the world.

Marc, recognizing the potential of myofunctional therapy in Europe, spent a significant amount of time there building connections and collaborations. His tireless efforts, combined with his multilingual skills and connections, allowed him to gain traction and make substantial progress. European countries, with their focus on public health and cost reduction, were particularly interested in implementing these therapies, especially for prenatal women with a history of sleep and breathing disorders. Countries like France, Italy, and Spain were investing in research, neurodevelopmental assessments, and outcome studies to understand the impact of these disorders on infants and their subsequent development.

The success of the congress and the growing interest in myofunctional therapy in Europe led to further initiatives and collaborations. Researchers were comparing the developmental milestones and movements of children with airway and sleep disorders to those without such conditions, revealing remarkable differences. In Spain, they were gathering outcome data to evaluate the effectiveness of treatments like myofunctional therapy and adenoid tonsillectomy.

It was fascinating to witness the impact of myofunctional therapy and the growing recognition of airway issues in prenatal care across different countries. The outcomes and ongoing studies were shedding light on the neurological implications and the need for early intervention in infants born with maxillary and mandibular anomalies, high arches, and retrusive chins. The dedication of professionals like Marc and the collaborative efforts of experts around the world were paving the way for a paradigm shift in prenatal care.

Through all these experiences, what struck me the most was the attention given to prenatal moms in Europe. They are recognizing that if a mother has sleep apnea or related issues, there's a high likelihood that their baby could develop similar issues. It's impressive how they are making strides to better understand and address these issues before they escalate.

The key here is early detection and intervention. Countries like Japan that evaluate these conditions from birth and begin treatments during toddlerhood see fewer complications.

What I discovered recently is the focus on the "First 1,000 Days" in Europe. They have conducted studies and events to understand how this critical period affects human performance throughout a lifetime. The term first one-thousand days refers to the period from conception until a child's second birthday. This critical period of growth and development lays the foundation for a person's future health, behavior, and intellectual capacity. The concept emphasizes the importance of optimal nutrition, healthcare, and nurturing during this period, as it profoundly influences a child's ability to grow, learn, and rise out of poverty, as well as their risk for disease in adulthood.

The first one-thousand days concept is widely recognized in fields like developmental biology, pediatric health, and public health. It's based on scientific research showing that proper nutrition during this period can secure a long-term health trajectory that extends into adulthood. It can prevent stunting, promote cognitive development, improve educational achievement, and even increase adult wages.

The first one-thousand days are divided into three key stages:

1. From conception until birth: Proper nutrition and healthcare for the pregnant mother directly impact the baby's development in the womb. Lack of certain nutrients can lead to birth defects or long-term health issues.

2. From birth until six months: Breastfeeding provides newborns with all the nutrients they need for healthy development during this stage. It also provides immunological protection and can impact future eating habits and preferences.

3. From six months to two years: This period is characterized by rapid growth and the introduction of solid foods. Proper nutrition during this stage is critical for continued growth and cognitive development.

It's during these one-thousand days that a child's brain develops most rapidly, and nutrition, along with nurturing care and stimulation, plays a significant role in this process. Providing optimal nutrition and care during this window has a substantial impact on a child's ability to grow, learn, and thrive.

Airway health disorders are a global concern, and various countries are taking preventive measures to address this issue. Many parents, especially in the United States, might not be fully aware of the advancements other countries have made in managing airway health conditions. While the specific approaches may vary, the overarching goal is to promote optimal airway health and reduce the prevalence of related conditions. Here are some examples of what other countries are doing in this regard:

- **United Kingdom (U.K.):** The U.K. places significant emphasis on raising awareness about airway health disorders, particularly in children.

Initiatives such as the National Health Service's (NHS) Healthy Child Programme focus on educating parents and caregivers about the importance of maintaining a healthy airway and providing guidance on appropriate interventions. Additionally, the NHS promotes regular dental check-ups for children to detect and address any early signs of airway-related issues.

- **Australia:** In Australia, there is increasing recognition of the impact of airway health disorders on overall well-being. Dental and medical professionals collaborate to assess and manage these conditions. The Australian Society of Orthodontists emphasizes early orthodontic intervention to optimize airway development in children. There is also ongoing research and public health campaigns raising awareness about the importance of nasal breathing, proper oral posture, and healthy lifestyle habits.

- **Sweden:** Sweden has a proactive approach to airway health, particularly in relation to sleep-disordered breathing. The Swedish public health system provides comprehensive healthcare services, including early diagnosis and treatment of sleep apnea and other airway-related conditions. Specialized sleep clinics and multidisciplinary teams work together to assess and manage these disorders effectively.

- **Brazil:** Brazil has implemented national programs aimed at promoting airway health. The Brazilian Ministry of Health has developed initiatives focusing on early detection and intervention for children with airway disorders, including regular assessments and treatment plans. Furthermore, public health campaigns and educational programs raise awareness among healthcare professionals and the general public about the importance of airway health. About a decade ago, Brazil implemented an infant frenulum inspection nationwide to identify potential airway issues at birth. Results continue to be tabulated and evaluated.

- **Singapore:** Singapore places a strong emphasis on preventive measures for airway health disorders, particularly in pediatric care. The Ministry of Health in Singapore encourages early detection of conditions such as obstructive sleep apnea, providing guidelines for healthcare professionals on screening and appropriate interventions. Public health education campaigns promote healthy lifestyle habits and encourage regular dental check-ups to maintain optimal airway health.

- **Finland:** Finland has been recognized for its comprehensive approach to airway health and prevention of breathing-related issues in infants. The Finnish Maternity Package, a government initiative, provides expectant mothers with a baby box containing essential items, including a mattress that promotes safe sleeping positions and helps prevent positional skull deformities.

- **Netherlands:** In the Netherlands, the "Dutch Approach" focuses on prenatal and postnatal care to promote healthy airway development in infants. This approach emphasizes breastfeeding, correct positioning during sleep, and avoiding exposure to tobacco smoke. Additionally, the Netherlands actively promotes research and education on airway health disorders.

- **Japan:** In Japan, there is a strong emphasis on educating parents about airway health and prevention of issues such as positional skull deformities and sleep-related breathing disorders. Dr. Abe in Japan is also dedicated to improving toddlers' development, ensuring they can thrive academically. The Japanese Ministry of Health, Labour, and Welfare provides guidelines and resources to promote safe sleeping environments for infants.

While the U.S. has made significant strides in managing airway health disorders, there is much to learn from global practices. Emphasizing prevention, utilizing technology, implementing public health campaigns, and driving policy reforms are strategies that have shown promise in other countries. Parents can take a proactive role by understanding these approaches and incorporating relevant strategies into their children's health management.

In the U.S., doctors and hospitals tend to treat an asthma attack without adequately managing the triggers that cause the attacks, for example.

Australia is leading the way in employing technology to manage airway disorders. The National Asthma Council of Australia endorses smart inhalers, which offer real-time data to clinicians, allowing them to evaluate and adjust the treatment as needed [3]. While smart inhalers are also available in the U.S., they are not as widely used or known among parents. Incorporating this technology can give parents a more accurate picture of their child's condition, offering insights into when and why symptoms worsen and how effective the treatment is.

Finland has implemented an innovative national allergy program aimed at reducing allergy-related public health issues and healthcare costs. The program uses a comprehensive approach involving prevention, early diagnosis, and efficient care. Through public awareness campaigns, parents are educated about managing allergies and asthma, recognizing symptoms, and understanding when to seek medical help. This contrasts with the United States' approach, where public health campaigns on airway disorders are not as comprehensive and parents are left to research information on their own.

In the U.S., the National Heart, Lung, and Blood Institute (NHLBI) has developed guidelines for the diagnosis and management of asthma, emphasizing coordinated care across healthcare providers. While the guidelines are a step in the right direction, they are not always fully implemented in healthcare practice.

In comparison, many European countries have implemented more consistent nationwide strategies for managing airway disorders. These strategies involve not just individual healthcare providers but also schools, workplaces, and other community organizations, creating a more comprehensive support network for individuals with these conditions.

In Japan, combating airway disorders has become a national priority due to its aging population. Japan has an extensive home healthcare system to cater to patients with chronic conditions like chronic obstructive pulmonary disease (COPD). Home-visit nursing, physical therapy, and respiratory care are made available to the elderly and those who cannot easily visit a hospital.

Moreover, Japanese healthcare policy provides for preventive healthcare services, which include routine screenings, preventive guidance, and health education. The goal is to catch health problems early before they become chronic or severe [7]. By adopting similar practices, American families could potentially lower the incidence of severe airway disorders by focusing on early detection and intervention.

Countries with universal healthcare systems, like the United Kingdom, Canada, and many in the European Union, often cover preventive services in their health plans. This is based on the understanding that early detection and intervention can prevent more serious health problems down the line, ultimately saving costs.

In contrast, the U.S. healthcare system often focuses more on treating disease than preventing it. The majority of healthcare costs go toward treating chronic diseases, many of which are preventable. While some health insurance plans do cover preventive services, they may be underutilized due to lack of awareness or high deductibles and copayments.

For those dependent on Medicaid, the terrain is particularly tricky. Coverage is a patchwork that varies state by state, often limited to fundamental treatments like CPAP machines for sleep apnea. More holistic or preventive treatments such as myofunctional therapy may fall outside of Medicaid's purview. Recognizing the constraints of your Medicaid benefits can be the key to crafting alternative routes for adequate care.

If you're dealing with private insurance, prepare yourself for a bureaucratic odyssey. Billing codes are often not intuitive, and claims for what insurance companies deem "experimental" or "non-essential" treatments may be swiftly denied. Your best defense is to arm yourself with knowledge: discuss billing codes directly with your healthcare provider and mount appeals against denials when necessary.

Worst of all, many airway health services are not covered by insurance, forcing families to pay out of pocket and increasing costs for the help that their children need. This puts undue hardship on families who may not be able to afford the treatment their children need.

Sixty-two percent of all personal bankruptcies filed in the U.S. in 2007 were caused by medical problems—seventy-eight percent of those who filed had medical insurance, at least at the start of their illness.[2]

According to Dr. Richard T. Seymour, "Health insurance companies should not have the right to exclude coverage of the chief sensory nerve of the head and face and a joint that is needed to speak, eat, digest, breathe, sleep, and for intimacy."[3]

In 2016, Blue Cross Blue Shield of Texas read my lengthy report on Savvy's orthognathic surgery and why it should be covered by our health insurance plan with them. The committee in charge of our claim also spoke with Dr. Larry Wolford about the necessity. Clearly, the surgery was lifesaving, and the claim was paid.

Insurance or not, the out-of-pocket costs of treating airway disorders can be substantial. From advanced sleep studies to orthodontic work and ongoing myofunctional therapy, the financial toll can quickly mount. Many families leverage Health Savings Accounts (HSAs) or Flexible Spending Accounts (FSAs) as a cushion, but even so, affordability often remains an elusive goal for quality care.

Confronted with these financial and systemic gaps, the role of advocacy becomes ever more pivotal. Grassroots campaigns, collaboration with nonprofits, and partnerships with medical professionals can amplify the call for change, helping to push the needle on how airway health is funded and addressed in both the public and private sectors.

It's important for parents to understand their health insurance coverage and advocate for necessary preventive services to be covered for their children. By focusing on prevention, it's possible to detect and manage airway disorders early, potentially preventing more severe health issues down the line. We'll talk about some other ways to cover funding in the next section.

TEN
ADVOCATING FOR YOUR CHILD

"Your child's adult health-span (the number of healthy years a person can live into old age) depends on how we approach these issues today. I live in the trenches of advanced airway disorders and it's wretched. It should freak us out that an estimated 26% of Americans have obstructive sleep apnea (OSA) today... and only 4% have been diagnosed." [1]

-AN EXCERPT FROM *BRAVE PARENT* BY DR. SUSAN MAPLES, DDS, MSBA

Recently, a young family reached out to me with concerns about their ten-year-old son, who was diagnosed with ADHD. He was being medicated with stimulants and having difficulty in school. Their dentist told them that their son had very narrow jaws, so they tried an upper palate expander. The expander kept coming out and was not working well for this child. They gave up. The dentist said that the child was not mature enough to keep the expander in.

We researched and found an expert airway-centric dentist in Phoenix. I reviewed the case studies and results of their other young patients and attended the first appointment with the family. The dentist explained that every case is unique. This child, who has very narrow jaws and an anterior tongue tie, would need to start with myofunctional therapy to help him adjust to upper and lower expanders. We all passed around the expanders and saw that they were supple and malleable, able to be removed for meals and set times during the day. Mom and Dad were shown how they could best support their son during his short daily myofunctional exercises, deal with concerns along the way, and reinforce good habits during the eight-to-ten-month process. The dentist recommended, if needed, an evaluation from an ENT to check adenoids and tonsils after the expansion process was underway, as the expansion process often reduces the inflammation of tonsils and adenoids. The ENT would also be involved in releasing the tongue tie after the expansion was completed so there would be room for the tongue to rest in its proper position of up and forward. Images were taken so the customized maxillary and mandibular expanders could be ordered. I noted that this family had a one-time lifetime orthodontic benefit with Blue Cross Blue Shield, which was applied to the overall cost.

At one point, this apprehensive and very energetic boy started to object. I sat down on the floor next to the exam table and told him about another boy I had met going through the same thing in Chicago with Dr. Kevin Boyd. His upper palate was expanded ten millimeters, and he could breathe, sleep, concentrate, and focus better than ever. In fact, he was standing on the exam table during his final appointment, jumping up and down so excited about how well he would now be able to play little league baseball! "I'll even be able to run faster!" he exclaimed. I assured him and his parents that some days might be kind of tough, but he was going to be able to think better, feel better, and do much better in school and sports.

We recently learned that the boy in Phoenix got his first straight-A report card after only six months of expansion and advancement treatment together with myofunctional exercises. (Before he started his treatment six months earlier, the school had recommended special ed classes because he couldn't focus!) Absolutely amazing. I'm so proud of his accomplishments and his parents' dedicated help and support.

To find airway-centric physicians, dentists, and allied providers in your area, please see www.childrensairway first.org.

When our children need vital medical care, almost inevitably there are significant financial concerns. Our commitment to our daughter's health was so strong that the company Brad works for once chose to renew their employee healthcare plan and benefits based on Savvy's needs. We were amazed! I remember meeting a mom in a waiting room who had sold several horses in order to get the care her daughter needed. Others told me that they would be working more years than they had planned to. I can't help thinking about the countless parents who may not have the same resources, so I am including examples of a few possibilities that I hope are inspiring and helpful for others.

I once suggested to my friend, whose son had leukemia, to consider the top three choices for his treatment. To my surprise, she hesitated, not wanting to disrupt her husband's career. Later, his boss, a friend of ours, reassured them, offering to cover all expenses if they wished to go to Boston for treatment. They even had the option to go to St. Jude's for free.

Another case was that of my best friend, who was diagnosed with oral cancer. Despite her initial reluctance to inconvenience her family, I finally convinced her that her family wanted her around and it was worth any sacrifice to help her heal. She ended up in a trial at Johns Hopkins, which happily extended her life by two and a half years.

Life circumstances should not stop us from being able to help us or our children with medically related conditions, no matter what.

Our mission through the Children's Airway First Foundation is to create awareness, provide resources, and foster conversations around airway disorders and their profound impact on children's lives. I want to provide guidance and support to parents who find themselves in overwhelming situations. It's crucial to have accessible information and resources available because, without them, families can feel stuck and helpless. We often connect parents with doctors and information, but what if they can't physically access the necessary care? It's an ongoing concern.

Another resource is United Way's 211 Helpline. They assist families and individuals with serious health conditions by arranging flights to the best hospitals and even covering expenses for the entire family. I called the service for a friend of mine a few years ago and said, "Her dad works for UPS, and they told me to call you because UPS decided to give all their money for family healthcare exceptions to your program. This girl has hEDS and a vascular disorder." United Way said, "Okay, we will fly her mom, her siblings, and the patient to Cincinnati because they have one of the best programs for her particular issue. We will pay for their babysitters, meals, lodging, etc. We can help them make all the arrangements and pay for everything." United Way's 211 service is there for a reason, so use it if you need it.

Additionally, starting a GoFundMe campaign can rally support from friends, family, and even strangers. I remember a case where a young girl with hEDS received significant financial aid—ten thousand dollars in two days—through a GoFundMe campaign, enabling her to seek treatment at a specialized facility.

Another powerful example is St. Jude's, where a family's six-year-old son received one hundred percent free care for his leukemia. They prioritize saving children's lives regardless of their ability to pay, as should be done in this country. There are organizations prioritizing the care that needs to take place no matter what, and it's important to know what's available for your specific situation.

In all these stories and experiences, one thing remains clear: as parents, our primary aim is to ensure the best for our children, even if it means fighting against odds. The critical part is to keep searching for the right help and resources, even when the path seems challenging and overwhelming.

One of the absolute best resources you can turn to when you need help for your child is the *U.S. News & World Report*, where it ranks the best hospitals by department speciality. If you're giving birth to a child with an obvious breathing disorder, or you can see in utero skeletal dysplasia happening, Children's National in Washington, D.C., has the number one neonatology unit in the whole country. If you want to be cured of cancer, go to MD Anderson. They have a ninety-nine percent cure rate. They're number one in adults, but number twenty-two in children. Where do you go if you have a child with leukemia? The top three are usually Children's Hospital of Philadelphia, St. Jude's in Memphis, or Boston Children's. The report will also show you the rating for each.

Each hospital's rankings in different specialties, such as heart surgery or gastroenterology, vary significantly. It is essential to consider these rankings when making decisions about medical care.

When you are searching for a healthcare professional who

can best help you with knowledge and expertise in airway health, consider asking the following questions.

1. **Can you explain your experience with airway health disorders?** Knowing about the healthcare provider's past experience with diagnosing and treating airway disorders can give you a sense of their knowledge and competence.

2. **What diagnostic tests do you typically use to evaluate airway disorders?** A comprehensive approach typically involves a variety of tests like spirometry, imaging studies, and sleep studies. Asking this question can provide insight into their diagnostic process.

3. **What treatment options do you commonly use for managing airway disorders?** The response to this question can show you whether the provider is familiar with the range of treatments, from lifestyle changes to medications, orthodontic treatments, and surgery.

4. **Can you explain your approach to developing a personalized treatment plan?** A good healthcare provider should take a holistic view of the patient, considering all aspects of their health, lifestyle, and personal circumstances when developing a treatment plan.

5. **What other doctors, teams, or resources do you work with in developing the treatment plan?** This will let you know if they place importance on

multidisciplinary teams to address what needs to take place.

6. **How often do you typically follow up with patients during the treatment process?** Regular follow-ups are essential for monitoring progress and adjusting the treatment plan as necessary.

7. **Are you familiar with the latest research and developments in the field of airway health disorders?** Medicine is a constantly evolving field. The provider's awareness of current research can give you a sense of their commitment to keeping their knowledge updated.

8. **Can you provide references or testimonials from other patients you've treated with airway health disorders?** Hearing about the experiences of other patients can offer valuable insights into the healthcare provider's expertise and patient care philosophy.

Remember, it is important to have open and transparent communication with healthcare professionals to ensure that your child's airway health is thoroughly assessed and addressed. Don't hesitate to ask follow-up questions or seek a second opinion if needed. Your active involvement and advocacy as a parent can make a significant difference in your child's overall well-being.

I know I've repeated myself a few times through this, but it's because there is such an immense task ahead of us to comprehend this, and we don't have time to lose. It's like realizing my child, whose ankles are so weak they keep turning, is losing her memory. She used to be one of the brightest kids, and suddenly something is off. Yet the observation from others is, "She has become quite lazy," instead of recognizing that something's fundamentally wrong. The comments turn from concern to judgment: "She's not trying anymore; maybe there are issues at home? Are her parents getting divorced? Is there abuse?" And while these concerns are well-intentioned, they're missing the point, the crucial clues, such as, "Why are her fingernails turning blue?" Sadly, I didn't notice this either, even though I saw her every day. She was always so pale, and the bluish tint seemed normal for her.

Looking back to her early years, her first and second grade teachers didn't want to embarrass her. She was a bright, charming student with a malocclusion that made her teeth stand out like a cartoon. She had only one friend with a similar issue, and the rest of the kids seemed to alienate her. Retractive braces are part of our culture these days. Many people don't understand that the things deemed normal are actually severely hurting our children. If a dentist wants to pull teeth and apply retractive orthodontics, run! Most likely the mouth will end up shrinking, resulting in a lifetime of breathing disorders and the comorbidities so common to those with sleep apnea.

The most frustrating part is that all of these issues could have been corrected when she was an infant. It's not widely understood how the growth of your jaws can affect your entire body. For instance, we've been helping Savvy's boyfriend, who grew up in a foster home, restore his mouth. His former dentist installed stainless steel crowns on his molars that were too high, causing him constant headaches and chewing and swallowing problems. Once these were removed and he received a temporary restoration, the headaches stopped. He had lived with the pain, medicating with six to eight aspirins a day, wreaking havoc on his digestive system. He could have been saved from all of this.

However, like for many of us, understanding this "new approach" wasn't easy for him. We had to explain it to him. But seeing and feeling the impact of the treatment, he expressed profound gratitude. He was so appreciative, thanking us profusely and calling us a "gift to humanity."

One evening, he noticed a book under my coffee table about ADHD and ADD called *Stolen Focus* by Yuhan Hari. He mentioned how he struggles with focus and gets easily distracted. We handed him the book, hoping it might help him understand his challenges better.

Consider how many children and adults are diagnosed with ADD, ADHD, and similar disorders. What if these issues stem from an airway or sleep disorder? This could explain why they struggle with everyday tasks like homework or sitting in a classroom for hours and why they read a page and can't recall what they've just read.

We know as parents when there's something wrong. Sometimes it's easier to turn a blind eye or trust the "professionals" over our gut, but I want to encourage you to not stop asking why until you have the real answers—not just a bandage for the symptom. Without the truth, our kids can endure years of emotional and physical pain that they shouldn't have to go through.

Here are some practical ways to advocate for your child's health in a school setting:

- **Identify the Issue:** Before approaching educators, understand the symptoms and complications related to your child's airway health. This knowledge provides credibility and urgency when you're making requests.

- **Engage the Right Personnel:** Start with the teacher, but don't hesitate to escalate the issue to the school nurse, counselor, or even the principal if needed.

- **Request Accommodations:** Whether it's more frequent breaks, a quieter classroom setting, or even a 504 plan for medical accommodations, know what could benefit your child and ask for it.

- **Educational Advocacy:** Share informative materials about airway health with school staff. The more they understand the issue, the better they can accommodate and support your child.

Here are some practical ways to advocate for your child's health in the healthcare setting:

- **Choose a Provider Wisely:** Look for healthcare providers familiar with airway health issues. A specialist is often more equipped to diagnose and treat these conditions.

- **Be Prepared:** Before medical appointments, make a list of symptoms, concerns, and any questions you might have.

- **Ask for Second Opinions:** If the proposed treatment doesn't feel right or sufficient, seek a second opinion. Trust your parental instincts.

- **Coordinated Care:** For multifaceted treatment approaches, make sure all healthcare providers involved are communicating and coordinating with each other. This includes dentists, orthodontists, and any therapists involved in your child's care.

Advocacy extends to dealing with insurance companies as you navigate finances. Know your rights and coverage details, and be prepared to appeal if a necessary treatment is denied. Sometimes a well-worded letter from a healthcare provider can tip the scales in your favor.

Another aspect of supporting your child is building a support network. Consider connecting with other families dealing with similar challenges. Support groups, whether online or in your community, can offer valuable advice and emotional support.

One of the best things you can do is empower your child as they grow, teaching them how to advocate for themselves. Understanding their condition and needs will enable them to seek help when you're not around.

Parents have an essential role to play in advocating for their children and driving change in their communities. By sharing their experiences and raising awareness, they can make a significant difference. Parents should establish collaborative relationships with their child's healthcare providers, including pediatricians, dentists, myofunctional therapists, and ENT specialists. Open communication, active engagement, and sharing relevant information can foster a team-based approach to addressing airway health disorders effectively. Exploring avenues for involvement and understanding the best practices employed by renowned institutions will empower parents to take action and create positive change for their children and others.

When it comes to addressing airway disorders within their own family, parents can take the following actions:

1. **Educate Yourself:** Gain knowledge about airway disorders in children. Understand the potential signs, symptoms, and risk factors associated with these conditions. Educate yourself about the

importance of proper airway health and its impact on overall well-being. I also have a list of resources to learn from in the back of this book.

2. **Observe and Assess Your Child:** Pay close attention to their child's breathing patterns, sleep quality, and overall behavior. Look for signs of mouth breathing, snoring, restless sleep, frequent awakenings, bedwetting, daytime sleepiness, and behavioral issues. Document any concerns or observations to discuss with healthcare professionals.

3. **Consult with Healthcare Professionals:** Schedule appointments with pediatricians, dentists, orthodontists, or other relevant healthcare providers to discuss your child's airway health. Ask specific questions about their assessment methods, experience with airway disorders, and any recommended screenings or evaluations. Parents must be aware of the diagnostic challenges associated with airway health disorders. Many medical professionals may not have sufficient training or awareness to detect these conditions early on. By understanding the limitations and potential gaps in current diagnostic practices, parents can advocate for improved screening protocols and training opportunities for healthcare providers.

4. **Seek a Multidisciplinary Approach:** Consider involving a team of professionals, including pediatricians, dentists, orthodontists, and ENT specialists, who can collaborate to assess and

manage your child's airway health comprehensively. Seek referrals or recommendations from healthcare professionals as needed.

5. **Implement Healthy Lifestyle Habits:** Promote practices that support optimal airway health in your family. Encourage proper nutrition, regular physical activity, good oral hygiene, and adequate sleep hygiene. Limit exposure to environmental allergens, irritants, and secondhand smoke.

6. **Foster Nasal Breathing:** Encourage nasal breathing in your child. Promote good nasal hygiene, such as using saline nasal sprays or rinses to keep the nasal passages clear. Teach your child techniques for breathing through the nose and provide gentle reminders when mouth breathing is observed.

7. **Maintain a Clean Sleeping Environment:** Create a sleep-friendly environment that minimizes potential allergens, dust, and pollutants. Use hypoallergenic bedding, regularly clean the bedroom, and consider investing in air purifiers to improve air quality.

8. **Support Healthy Oral Development:** Encourage proper oral posture and swallowing techniques in your child. Discourage thumb sucking or prolonged pacifier use, as these habits can impact oral and facial development. Consider consulting with a pediatric dentist or orthodontist who is knowledgeable about airway health.

9. **Promote Good Sleep Habits:** Establish consistent bedtime routines and ensure your child is getting enough quality sleep. Encourage a regular sleep schedule and create a calming environment that promotes relaxation before bedtime.

10. **Advocate for Airway Health:** Be an advocate for your child's airway health within the healthcare system. If you suspect an airway disorder is being overlooked or not taken seriously, seek a second opinion or consult with specialists who have expertise in this area. Don't accept the answer of "that's normal" or "they will grow out of it." Stay informed, ask questions, and actively participate in decisions regarding your child's healthcare. Parents play an active role in raising awareness about airway health disorders within their communities, schools, and healthcare settings. Organizing educational workshops, distributing informational materials, and sharing personal stories educate others and foster a greater understanding of these conditions. Parents can also actively participate in research initiatives focused on airway health disorders. By partnering with researchers, sharing their experiences, and contributing to data collection, parents can help drive evidence-based practices and advance knowledge in the field.

We have the power to advocate for policy changes that support early detection, appropriate diagnosis, and effective management of airway health disorders. By engaging with policymakers, attending public hearings, and sharing our experiences, we can influence the development of guidelines and regulations that prioritize children's airway health.

Looking back, I realize that all of this could have been prevented. If Savvy had been screened, evaluated, and treated before the age of four, she wouldn't have needed retractive braces. Her jaws would have been gently and non-surgically brought forward using manual manipulation or small dental implements, and her palate expanded to create enough space for all thirty-two teeth and proper tongue posture. Her nasopharynx complex would have been treated as well, teaching her to breathe through her nose and keep her mouth closed. She may not have had hypoxic brain injuries or struggled. She may not have felt like she was rotting away.

That's why I feel compelled to share our story with you. I never want you and your child to go through what we have been through. By sharing just a bit of the mounds of information I've discovered since, I want to make sure that every single parent is aware if their child is exhibiting relatable symptoms and is able to take the steps necessary toward the care needed for your child, protecting their future.

Today, Savvy is an articulate, composed, and intelligent individual who commands attention with her grace. I'm incredibly proud of her journey and her spirit, an embodiment of strength, intelligence, and resilience. I will just never be able to give her the health she should have had from the beginning or restore the time lost as we searched for answers.

Imagine a reality where airway health is no longer a puzzle but rather a fundamental consideration in pediatric care. Where parents have access to the tools and knowledge required to ensure their children breathe safely and sleep soundly. Where childhood development is supported rather than stymied by airway and sleep disorders. Our children deserve nothing less.

Remember, your child deserves a happier, healthier life. As James Nestor, the author of *Breath: The New Science of a Lost Art,* says, "There is nothing more essential to our health and well-being than breathing."[2] An aware parent is an empowered parent. By working together, we can ensure our children's health is prioritized and not overlooked. The future of our children is quite literally in our hands. As a parent or caregiver, you are the first line of defense in ensuring that your child receives the appropriate care and accommodations they need for their airway health disorder. Your advocacy shapes not just your child's health but also helps educate the institutions and systems you interact with, creating a more understanding and informed environment for all. Let's ensure they breathe and sleep easily and grow up healthy and strong. The path to prevention and cure begins with awareness. Let's spread the word and make the invisible visible.

It's time to break the silence around the silent pandemic and prioritize airway health, for every breath we take is a measure of our quality of life. Our children's quality of life depends on it.

DR. JOHN R. FINNEGAN AND SHARON MOORE - THE CRISIS OF AIRWAY HEALTH

Children's Airway Health as a Public Health Challenge

By John R. Finnegan Jr., PhD
Dean & Professor Emeritus, University of Minnesota
and
Sharon Moore
Speech Pathologist & Myofunctional Practitioner

"When health is absent, wisdom cannot reveal itself, art cannot become manifest, strength cannot fight, wealth becomes useless, and intelligence cannot be applied."

HEROPHILUS OF CHALCEDON, 335-280 BCE

"Man's mind, once stretched by a new idea, never regains its original dimensions."

OLIVER WENDELL HOLMES

Estimates are that hundreds of millions of children worldwide experience impaired airways and breathing. This places them at greater developmental risk, affecting sleep patterns, intellectual ability, behavior, and quality of life.[1] Correctable craniofacial syndromes are among the root causes yet can be complicated and amplified by connective tissue disorders[2], poverty, toxic air pollution, poor indoor air, and more.[3]

Unobstructed breathing and sleep are critical to health, an insight known since ancient times. Today, we also know that they are key to brain development as an infant, child, and adolescent because they form the basis for full adult functioning. This realm of knowledge, insight, and practice is experiencing a renewal in our sleep-deprived 21st century. Nestor's 2020 book *Breath*, co-author Moore's 2019 *Sleep Wrecked Kids*, and Walker's 2017 *Why We Sleep* are important examples of recent popular and scientific work.[4]

Problems of this magnitude and complexity move into the realm of "public health." But what does that entail? What are the modes of addressing such a complex problem? Who should lead, and who should be engaged? What strategies promote change? In this discussion, we focus on the challenge of preventing developmental disorders among children extending from correctable craniofacial syndromes and airway disorders that are physically at the root of so many. To begin, some basics about public health.

More than a century ago, the founding dean of the Yale School of Public Health, Charles E.A. Winslow, captured the purposes of public health as "...the science and art of preventing disease, prolonging life, and promoting human health [and well-being] through organized efforts and informed choices of society, public and private, organizations, communities, and individuals."

Much is embedded in this definition and provides a collective, collaborative framework that encompasses the responsibilities and obligations of public health and all the health professions in a connected arc of "prevention."[5]

The word itself comes from the Latin *praeventus*, which literally means to *anticipate* or *hinder*. In modern usage, prevention includes four levels:[6]

1) **"primordial prevention"** (changing "upstream" environmental and social conditions for whole populations that lead to "downstream" disease, illness, or infirmity). The preamble of the World Health Organization's (WHO) 1946 Constitution emphasized this point after World War II: "Health is a state of complete physical, mental, and social well-being and not merely the absence of disease or infirmity." Today, we understand this in terms of "social determinants of health" that contribute to long and healthy lives: living conditions, education, and work free of racism, discrimination, violence, poverty, addiction, and other factors known to shorten lives;[7]

2) **"primary prevention"** (strategies aimed at healthy individuals or populations to reduce risk exposure and maintain good health);

3) **"secondary prevention"** (focusing on early detection such as screening for conditions before they cause problems); and

4) **"tertiary prevention"** (focus on affected individuals to reduce the severity of the illness and any long-term impacts).

In this prevention framework, public health is about the collective "us" that includes populations, nations, and societies worldwide. Public health is the intersection of all the health sciences, professions, and all public and private sectors of the world, supporting health locally and across the globe and driving the politics to make it happen. This is especially so when the challenges we face are enormously complex. It should be "all hands on deck."

Reflecting on the experience of the 21st century, public health expert Edward F. Lawler and others have noted that "the complexity of public health and social problems is becoming more challenging. Understanding and designing solutions for these problems requires perspectives from multiple disciplines and fields as well as cross-disciplinary research and practice teams."[8]In other words, we must plan systematically and creatively about who should be at the table to help meet a public health challenge. What resources, perspectives, disciplines, powers, and influences are needed? Among the multitude of public health problems in the 21st century, one set of choices does not fit every challenge.

Making Effective Change: Process and "Why"

Addressing public health challenges in a complex world means first understanding the parameters of the situation and the "players": groups, institutions, and other forces that impinge on the problem yet may also prove necessary to engage in defining solutions.[9] The social ecological model has become standard in public health to help sort out the nature of public health problems, their manifestations, root causes, magnitude of impact on populations, and prospective actions necessary for remediation in complex settings.[10] Data plays a major role in scoping these dimensions, which in some cases may be in short supply when a public health challenge is emerging. In conjunction with the social ecological model, the theory of change model focuses on necessary and sufficient adaptive strategies and interventions to make a positive difference: awareness, education, use of technology, policy-making, collective action by engaged and powerful groups and institutions, and so on. This model forces an important discussion of the "what, how, and wherefores" of action for change and what to articulate as "success." Design thinking from multiple disciplines helps to format both intervention prototyping and dynamic adaptability in an ongoing iterative process.

"Gaps" in the chain of prevention and care include lack of knowledge of developmental risk among various groups: health professionals, policymakers, and parents themselves, for example. Former CDC Director Thomas Frieden summarized six components necessary for public health program effectiveness:[11]

(1) innovation to develop the statistical evidence for action;

(2) a technical package of a limited number of high-priority, evidence-based interventions that together will have a major impact;

(3) effective performance management, especially through rigorous, real-time monitoring, evaluation, and program improvement;

(4) partnerships and coalitions with public- and private-sector organizations;

(5) communication of accurate and timely information to the health care community, decision makers, and the public to affect behavior change and engage civil society; and

(6) political commitment to obtain resources and support for effective action.

Children's Airway First Foundation (CAFF)[12] was founded in 2021 to begin defining the challenge, what "change" looks like, and the pathways to effective achievement. Its vision statement is to "End the evolutionary pandemic of children's airway and sleep disorders." To achieve the vision, its mission is "to fix by six." To achieve both, some key questions for consideration are: why, what, who, how, and where to from here?

Simon Sinek, who coaches leadership in business, writes in *Starts with Why* that when people understand why, it shapes a compelling higher purpose that drives behaviour change and motivates people to think, act, and do things differently.[13]

"Why" tells us that there are few things more compelling than the voice of a mum or dad striving to end their child's suffering and to find solutions for their child's deteriorating condition, irrespective of access to the best health care in the country. On a global level, is there anything more compelling than knowing that more than four hundred million children globally suffer from breathing and sleep challenges that interfere with brain development and acquisition of developmental milestones, altering both health and education trajectories?[14] Yet, a high percentage of children under age six with breathing and sleep challenges and recognizable comorbidities remain unrecognized and untreated.

The need to promote sleep health in the global public health agenda was outlined by the World Sleep Society task force in 2023. Children, they stated, are particularly vulnerable to sleep deficiency, leading to behavior problems early in life. Childhood sleep deficiency is also associated with sleep deficiency in adulthood. And growing up in poverty or an otherwise unstable home environment predicts shorter sleep duration and a greater risk of breathing disturbances in children.[15]

The society's white paper on pediatric sleep, also published in 2023, reinforced that early diagnosis and treatment of obstructive sleep apnea (OSA) are critical, including identifying OSA risk factors such as secondhand smoke exposure, upper airway resistance syndrome, obesity, apnea of prematurity, and central OSA. They reinforced the requirement for precision treatment.[16,17]

OSA is one aspect of the spectrum of ventilatory disorders

impacting sleep, often labeled as sleep disordered breathing (SDB). Beyond OSA, snoring and other breathing disturbances can impact sleep efficacy even in the absence of hypoxia, with similar sequelae.[18,19] SDB is prevalent in children, and the earliest signs are measurable by medical, dental, and allied health specialists who assess the anatomic-physiological integrity of the upper airway. Such examination is key to identifying the aetiology of SDB.[20]

Research also reveals a developing burden of chronic disease associated with untreated SDB (especially OSA), yet not one health system globally is equipped to deal with the projected avalanche of chronic disease in aging populations.[21] The pathogenesis of OSA and other forms of SDB can be traced to childhood, conditions that children do not "grow out of."[22]

Altogether, a compelling "why" indeed!

Making Effective Change: What Needs to Happen?

As mentioned, data are important tools in creating change but also obviously not sufficient alone. To make it useful, data must be collected systemically and be available not only to health professionals and researchers but also to policymakers, families, childcare workers, and early education teachers and staff in the case of children's airway disorders. For the latter groups, data need to be framed in "digestible" formats that tell an important story that can be heard, understood, and accepted.[23] The good news at this writing is that there is more attention being paid to the need for data globally. One such recent effort (2021) gathered data across 68.7 million children, concluding that "early management of common comorbid conditions to SDB is key."[24] More systematically gathered data is needed, nevertheless. Yet, available research, alongside the voice of families whose children suffered in the past or currently from a lack of early intervention and healthcare, has helped mobilize "airway" health care professionals and parents. CAFF is a prominent voice in the movement to obtain better science and data and to articulate it for lay understanding and education.[25] In the case of valid and reliable data, a global problem ultimately requires a global solution through international collaborative networks led perhaps by the World Health Organization (WHO). In lieu of that, it makes sense to advocate for valid and reliable national efforts.[26]

Change and Public Policy

In a perfect world, lobbying the government to recognise the existence of gaps in the chain of pediatric health care, including the fiscal impacts of untreated pediatric airway and sleep challenges, should take center stage. Perhaps the burgeoning development of chronic disease in aging populations is a driving force? Perhaps the fiscal implications to governments, with an estimated cost of 1.5 percent GDP, are a driver amplifying the challenge's impact if nations do little or nothing? In public health, outcomes in prevention often follow a simple rule: "Invest in prevention now or expect enormous costs later." Benjamin Franklin said it more simply: "An ounce of prevention is worth a pound of cure. "It's a lesson human civilization has struggled with for centuries. Yet there is no doubt that airway and sleep disorders properly treated in children's earliest years would reduce healthcare costs and increase the availability of funds for other important national priorities.[27]

It's not easy to garner the attention of government bodies, yet in Australia, the Australasian Sleep Association and Sleep Health Foundation joined forces, lobbying Parliament relentlessly. The outcome was a national inquiry into the sleep health of Australians launched in 2019 and followed in 2023 by a Federal Department of Health commitment to support sleep as a pillar of health alongside nutrition and physical activity.[28] Although a public health campaign is not in the cards at this writing, education in sleep health will be fully integrated into existing health promotion campaigns. This is a triumph for the health of Australians and shows unequivocally that change is possible, especially through organized collective action.

While Europe and Australia have made progress, the public health challenge of children's airways is not high generally on the agenda of U.S. health professionals, policymakers, and, consequently, parents of newborns themselves. Consider the potential benefits of early diagnosis of impaired breathing in newborns. While every U.S. state requires newborn screening, there are none at this writing that include examination of the oral cavity or craniofacial anatomy with respect to impaired breathing.[29] Of course, craniofacial disorders such as cleft palate and certain infant lung dysfunction are obvious and require intervention. However, much less obvious but significant craniofacial variances often go undetected far past infancy or are missed entirely since they are not included in newborn screenings and appear to be overlooked in many early infant examinations.[30]

Although the U.S. Department of Health and Human Services (DHHS) provides a Recommended Uniform Screening Panel (RUSP), each state chooses what it will screen. RUSP currently makes no specific mention of examination of the oral cavity that may pose a cause of sleep disordered breathing (SDB) or other airway disorders. Unsurprisingly, no state requires it. Changing this most likely will require action in each state through departments of health and/or legislatures since U.S. states bear the major responsibility for public health and safety in the country. Although many organizations and health professionals seek mandated uniformity among the states, the history of infant screening over the past sixty years in the U.S. suggests that is unlikely any time soon without congressional intervention.[31]

The Role of the Health Professions, Practice, and Science

What are other options for introducing change to health-care beyond government policy?

National organizations such as the U.S. National Academy of Medicine (NAM) can be instrumental in building the scientific and statistical basis for needed change in health professional education and the problem of the country's hodgepodge of newborn screening panels. For example, an important NAM discussion paper authored by seven U.S. and European health professionals and scientists (2023) has called for nothing less than a transformation of the concept of oral health.[32] The importance of this document is the elevation of oral health from a "disease" model to a "health and well-being" model. It opens the door to deeper understanding of oral anatomy and physiology as crucial gateways to the development of human capabilities from infancy.

With respect to young children with breathing and sleep challenges, there is a difference between those with complex medical conditions and those otherwise healthy children. Clinically, their healthcare needs differ.[33] They do have things in common, however. Both groups require the structural and/or neuromuscular components of an airway problem to be "unravelled." It starts with screening. Newborn screening is an opportunity to recognise challenges as early as possible in a child's life. Every health care professional who has young children in their care has an opportunity to do a simple oral cavity or craniofacial structure examination with respect to dysfunctional breathing.[34]

In addition, the 67,000-member American Academy of Pediatrics (AAP) already recommends routine sleep screenings.[35] Newborn screening is an opportunity to recognise challenges as early as possible in a child's life. In lieu of official policy, "piggybacking" onto existing healthcare screening opportunities attended by children under age six is common sense. Expanding healthcare professionals' screening repertoire will require that they understand "why." This requires education and awareness in addition to reassessing medical and health science education.

To what extent are health professionals (e.g., dentists, physicians, and nurses) educated in the significance of children's airway disorders and have the practice skills for examination and diagnosis?

Perhaps adding standards of medical training reflected in primary care, pediatrics, and some specialty curricula may be needed.[36] Such an effort may require engaging education oversight institutions. For example, major curriculum changes in U.S. medical schools often come from the Liaison Committee for Medical Education (LCME) and the institutions that sponsor it: the American Association of Medical Colleges (AAMC), the American Medical Association (AMA), and the Accreditation Council for Graduate Medical Education (ACGME). The American Academy of Family Physicians (AAFP) also develops evidence from the research literature guiding clinical practice guidelines. In the education and training of dentists, it is the American Dental Association's (ADA) Commission on Dental Accreditation that fulfills this role. For schools and colleges of nursing, there are two independent bodies: the Accreditation Commission for Education in Nursing (ACEN) and the Commission on Collegiate Nursing Education (CCNE).

In the past two decades, there been substantial progress across the health professions in what has come to be called "interprofessional health education." This movement began in the late 1960s in the U.K. with a focus on greater collaboration across the health professions to improve primary and community care in general.[37] The movement did not start in earnest in the U.S. until the early 2000s but received an important boost in 2010 with congressional passage of the Patient Protection and Affordable Care Act. Organizations such as the Interprofessional Education Collaborative (IPEC) and the National Center for Interprofessional Practice and Education (NEXUS) have successfully pushed forward an agenda for health professional education in collaborative, patient-centered community and population-oriented practice and care.[38] The effort has resulted in curricular change in the areas of values, ethics, communication, teamwork and team-based care, and roles and responsibilities for collaborative practice. Medicine, for example, with its decades-long emphasis on a biomedical model of care, has struggled to recognize that 21st century health challenges require a public health approach that incorporates "upstream" social determinants as agents of disease causation. The seeds of change have been planted and are sprouting.[39]

In this changing environment of the health professions, it is also important to note that there are eminent practitioner "champions" with knowledge, practice, and experience in children's airway issues who, together, could be especially effective in raising its public profile and its prevention and proper care. Several serve on the CAFF board. More are needed.

Stakeholders: Teachers, Child Care Workers, and Parents

Every day, early childhood educators and childcare workers have a bird's eye view of the "fall out" of untreated airway and sleep disorders—learning, memory, focus and emotional regulation challenges, missed milestones, speech-language delays, and behaviour that can be misdiagnosed as ADHD. They see signs and symptoms of poor executive function that typify many children with airway and sleep challenges but may not understand the cause. They also may be unaware of the impact of airway disorders and the simple signs of breathing and upper airway disorders. Yet they are in a perfect position to observe children's behaviour up close every day, to fully inform parents, and to encourage them to seek professional help.

Parents are by far the most powerful storytellers because their strong voices resonate with parents everywhere. There is nothing quite as effective as the impassioned rant of a parent unable to find the proper care for their child, not for days or weeks, but for years. Melody Yazdani scripted a famous Facebook rant in October 2018 that was viewed more than 300,000 times. She apologized upfront for "yelling in writing."

"Children should not breathe through their mouth," she wrote. "Not while awake, not while asleep. Never... All the signs were there, yet we had no clue..." [40] This was despite visiting multiple medical specialists, being soundly dismissed, trialing medications, and enduring their young son's out-of-control behavior daily.

Social media can be a powerful and compelling platform for parents experiencing the challenges described by Melody and others. But parents also struggle with social media and wonder which are the credible sources they can turn to for help considering so much misinformation floods media platforms? How do parents know whose voice is credible, especially as they seek professional help?

In 2022, the popular singer Halsey shared a story of growing up with an undiagnosed airway disorder that made her "sick for a long time," until an initial diagnosis in 2022 as an adult.[41] Along the way, the singer was labelled "crazy and lazy," given every diagnosis except the correct one, causing years of avoidable suffering.

Yet such change at the local level need not wait for a

slower-moving national effort. Change efforts at the state level could include drafting a model statute or administrative rule for an oral cavity exam, backed by a strong coalition of health professionals and parent-teacher organizations. Each of these groups most often observes and directly experiences the results of obstructive sleep apnea and other outcomes engendered by children's impaired breathing. They can make the most compelling case that catching the condition early impacts both health care and various education costs downstream, let alone the prospect of enhancing healthy, productive, and creative lives.

Postscript

There are many public health success stories over the decades.[42] Nearly all have required understanding root causes of the challenges addressed, creative design of potential solutions and strategies, building and sustaining community coalitions of public and private sector representatives who can influence, promote, and effect change, and access to resources. They require long-term commitment, especially if desired outcomes involve behavior, public policy change, or adoption of new technology or frameworks of understanding, or all the aforementioned. Those that succeed usually have carefully designed information feedback loops that indicate what is or isn't working and why. This permits "course correction," jettison or reconfiguration of strategies where necessary, and continuous adaptation to changing conditions.

Finally, among the important lessons learned from public health successes and failures is that communication in the digital age of social media is quite different from the analog world many of us were born into.[43] In the analog era of public health campaigns, media communication was generally one-way, or at best, facilitated delayed feedback. Social media did not yet exist which today permits immediate interaction, the creation of isolating echo chambers, and powerful networks filled with misinformation at best or devoted to spreading outright disinformation at worst. The recent experience of public health and the COVID-19 pandemic is a case in point.

We believe that the most successful public health communicators engaged the public factually, truthfully, and without arrogance, yet with the humility to say, "There is so much we don't yet know. Please bear with us as we learn," or words to that effect. Words matter, especially in polarized societies where all is "politicized," experts as well as the institutions they inhabit are suspect elites, and civil discourse is increasingly sparse. In this environment, public trust is easily lost and hard to regain.

In this environment, we also believe an alignment of "champions" among health care professionals, education professionals, and parents is capable of a compelling storytelling synergy that stimulates public interest, knowledge, empathy, and even trust. These are important ingredients for raising the challenge of children's airway health higher on the public agenda and cultivating persuasive grounds for change.

REFERENCES

INTRODUCTION

1. Tan HL, Kheirandish-Gozal L, Abel F, Gozal D. Craniofacial syndromes and sleep-related breathing disorders. Sleep Med Rev. 2016 Jun; 27:74-88. doi: 10.1016/j.smrv.2015.05.010. Epub 2015 Jun 6. PMID: 26454241; PMCID: PMC5374513. See also National Scientific Council on the Developing Child (2020 June), Connecting the Brain to the Rest of the Body: Early Childhood Development and Lifelong Health are Deeply Intertwined, Working Paper 15 (Retrieved from www.developingchild.harvard.edu. Center on the Developing Child, Harvard University, Cambridge, MA
2. Moore, Sharon, "*SleepWrecked Kids: Helping Parents Raise Happy, Health Kids, One Sleep at a Time*" 2020, Morgan James Publishing, Pgs. 21-22
3. Airway and Sleep Group. (n.d.). *The impact of mouth breathing on oral & general health*. https://airwayandsleepgroup.com/blog/the-impact-of-mouth-breathing-on-oral-general-health/
4. Sharon Moore, Sleep Wrecked Kids: Helping Parents Raise Happy, Healthy, Kids (Morgan Jarnes Publishing, 2020)

1. AIRWAY HEALTH AND THE URGENCY OF NOW

1. Leila Kheirandish-Gozal, 'Morbidity of OSA in Children', World Sleep Society Conference (Prague, 2017)
2. Walker, M. (2017). *Why we sleep: The new science of sleep and dreams*. Scribner.
3. Harper, R. M., Kumar, R., & Macey, P. M. (2012). Obstructive sleep apnea alters brain tissue concentrations of neurotransmitters and can lead to brain injury in children. *American Journal of Respiratory and Critical Care Medicine, 186*(8), 804-810. Retrieved from https://www.atsjournals.org
4. American Academy of Sleep Medicine. (2016). *Consensus statement on the recommended amount of sleep for children and adolescents*. Retrieved from https://aasm.org/resources/pdf/pediatricsleepdurationconsensus.pdf
5. Centers for Disease Control and Prevention (CDC). (2021). *Insufficient sleep is a public health epidemic*. Retrieved from https://www.cdc.gov/features/dssleep/index.html
6. American Academy of Sleep Medicine. (n.d.). *New national indicator report details importance of prompt sleep apnea diagnosis and treatment.*

Retrieved from https://aasm.org/new-national-indicator-report-details-importance-prompt-sleep-apnea-diagnosis-treatment/
7. *APA Blogs*. Published September 28, 2023. Accessed January 1, 2025. https://www.psychiatry.org/news-room/apa-blogs/treating-sleep-prob lems-may-prevent-depression#:~:text=Insomnia%2C%20the%20-most%20common%20sleep,make%20sleep%20tracking%20more%20accessible
8. Gozal, David, Ham, Sandra A, Mokhlesi, Babak. Sleep Apnea and Cancer: Analysis of a Nationwide Population Sample. *NIH Library. Sleep Med.* 2016 Aug 1; 39(8):1493-1500. doi: 10.5665/sleep.6004. Accessed January 1, 2025. https://pmc.ncbi.nlm.nih.gov/articles/PMC4945307/

3. THE URGENCY OF MONITORING SLEEP AND BREATHING IN AGES 0-2

1. Volpe, J. J. (2019). Neurology of the Newborn (6th ed.). Elsevier.
2. Hassiotou, F., & Geddes, D. T. (2013). Immune components in human milk and their effects on the development of the infant's immune system. *Frontiers in Pediatrics, 1,* 36. https://doi.org/10.3389/fped.2013.00036
3. Arman, A., & Basha, S. (2018). Breastfeeding and its impact on the development of the oral cavity and face: A systematic review. *Journal of Clinical Pediatric Dentistry, 42*(6), 452-456. https://doi.org/10.17796/1053-4625-42.6.452

4. UNVEILING THE HIDDEN SIGNS FOR AGES 3-5

1. Mitchell, R. B., & Kelly, J. (2013). Prevalence of obstructive sleep apnea in children with habitual snoring. *Sleep Medicine Reviews, 17*(1), 29-37. https://doi.org/10.1016/j.smrv.2012.01.003
2. Arman, A., & Basha, S. (2022). The impact of mouth breathing on dento-facial development. *Frontiers in Public Health, 10,* 929165.
3. American Academy of Sleep Medicine. (n.d.). *Obstructive sleep apnea.* https://aasm.org/resources/factsheets/sleepapnea.pdf
4. Pereira, L., Monyror, J., Almeida, F. T., Almeida, F. R., & Guerra, E. (2023). Prevalence of adenoid hypertrophy: A systematic review and meta-analysis. *Sleep Medicine Reviews, 68,* 101679. https://doi.org/10.1016/j.smrv.2022.101679
5. Chervin, R. D., Archbold, K. H., Dillon, J. E., Pituch, K. J., Panahi, P., & Dahl, R. E. (2002). Inattention, hyperactivity, and symptoms of sleep-disordered breathing. *Pediatrics, 109*(3), 449-456. https://doi.org/10.1542/peds.109.3.449
6. Gozal, D., & Kheirandish-Gozal, L. (2012). Obstructive sleep apnea and the metabolic syndrome in children. *Journal of Clinical Sleep Medicine, 8*(3), 301-306. https://doi.org/10.5664/jcsm.1916

7. Gelfand, A. A., & Goadsby, P. J. (2013). Headache and comorbidity in children and adolescents. *The Journal of Headache and Pain, 14*(1), 79. https://doi.org/10.1186/1129-2377-14-79

5. NAVIGATING AIRWAY HEALTH FOR AGES 5-10

1. Grippaudo, C., Majorana, A., & Gatto, R. (2016). Association between oral habits, mouth breathing, and malocclusion in Italian preschoolers. *Acta Otorhinolaryngologica Italica, 36*(5), 370-375. https://doi.org/10.14639/0392-100X-1010

7. THE COMPOUNDING IMPACT OF AIRWAY DISORDERS

1. Demmler, J. C., Atkinson, M. D., Reinhold, E. J., Choy, E., & Lyons, R. A. (2019). Diagnosed prevalence of Ehlers-Danlos syndrome and hypermobility spectrum disorder in Wales, UK: A national electronic cohort study and case–control comparison. *BMJ Open, 9*(11), e031365. https://doi.org/10.1136/bmjopen-2019-031365
2. Danielson, M. L., Bitsko, R. H., Ghandour, R. M., Holbrook, J. R., Kogan, M. D., & Blumberg, S. J. (2018). Prevalence of parent-reported ADHD diagnosis and associated treatment among US children and adolescents, 2016. *Journal of Clinical Child & Adolescent Psychology, 47*(2), 199-212. https://doi.org/10.1080/15374416.2017.1417860

8. SYSTEMIC HEALTH AND MULTIDISCIPLINARY TEAMS

1. American Academy for Oral Systemic Health. (n.d.). *Relationship between oral health and systemic disease.* https://www.aaosh.org/connect/relationship-between-oral-health-and-systemic-disease
2. Amin, R., Somers, V. K., McConnell, K., Willging, P. R., Myer, C. M., Sherman, M., McPhail, G., Morgenthal, A., Fenchel, M., Bean, J., Kimball, T. R., Daniels, S. R., & Gozal, D. (2008). Activity-adjusted 24-hour ambulatory blood pressure and cardiac remodeling in children with sleep-disordered breathing. *Hypertension, 51*(3), 84-91. https://doi.org/10.1161/HYPERTENSIONAHA.107.104314

9. A PUBLIC HEALTH IMPERATIVE: FOCUS ON PREVENTION

1. Hall, S. M. (2017). *The seven tools of healing: Unlock your inner wisdom and live the life your soul desires.* Balboa Press.

2. Himmelstein, D. U., Thorne, D., Warren, E., & Woolhandler, S. (2008). Medical bankruptcy in the United States, 2007: Results of a national study. *The American Journal of Medicine, 122*(8), 741-746. https://doi.org/10.1016/j.amjmed.2008.05.013
3. Seymour, R. T. (2013). *Stop the headache*. CreateSpace Independent Publishing Platform.

10. ADVOCATING FOR YOUR CHILD

1. Maples, S. (2020). *Brave parent: Raising healthy, happy, confident kids in the modern world*. The Brave Parent.
2. Nestor, J. (2020). *Breath: The new science of a lost art*. Riverhead Books.

DR. JOHN R. FINNEGAN AND SHARON MOORE - THE CRISIS OF AIRWAY HEALTH

1. Tan HL, Kheirandish-Gozal L, Abel F, Gozal D. Craniofacial syndromes and sleep-related breathing disorders. Sleep Med Rev. 2016 Jun; 27:74-88. doi: 10.1016/j.smrv.2015.05.010. Epub 2015 Jun 6. PMID: 26454241; PMCID: PMC5374513. See also National Scientific Council on the Developing Child (2020 June), Connecting the Brain to the Rest of the Body: Early Childhood Development and Lifelong Health are Deeply Intertwined, Working Paper 15 (Retrieved from www.developingchild.harvard.edu. Center on the Developing Child, Harvard University, Cambridge, MA).
2. For example, Ehlers-Danlos Syndromes (EDS): https://medlineplus.gov/genetics/condition/ehlers-danlos-syndrome/
3. Aithal SS, Sachdeva I, Kurmi OP. Air quality and respiratory health in children. Breathe (Sheff). 2023 Jun;19(2):230040. doi: 10.1183/20734735.0040-2023. Epub 2023 Jun 13. PMID: 37377853; PMCID: PMC10292770.
4. Nestor James (2020) *Breath: The New Science of a Lost Art*, Riverhead Books, New York. Moore, Sharon, *Sleep Wrecked Kids: Helping Parents Rise Happy, Healthy Kids One Sleep at a Time*, Morgan James Publishing, New York. Walker, Matthew, PhD, *Why We Sleep: Unlocking the Power of Sleep and Dreams*, Scribner, New York.
5. Advances in interprofessional collaboration and training among the health professions especially in the 21st Century also make clear that all health professions share in public health roles, responsibilities and obligations. This also has historical roots. See: Simon Finger (2012) *The Contagious City: The Politics of Public Health in Early Philadelphia*. Ithaca NY: Cornell University Press.
6. See Kisling, LA, Das, JM (2023), *Prevention Strategies*, US National Library of Medicine: https://www.ncbi.nlm.nih.-

gov/books/NBK537222/ Some add a 5th level focusing on "over-treatment."

7. Healthy People 2030, U.S. Dept of Health & Human Services (USDHH), Office of Disease Prevention & Health Promotion (OASH), Washington DC. https://health.gov/healthypeople. See also National Academies of Science, Engineering & Medicine (2020), *Leading Health Indicators 2030: Advancing Health, Equity and Well-Being* (Washington DC: NASEM).

8. Edward F. Lawler, PhD, Professor and Dean Emeritus, Brown School, Washington University, St Louis, Mo. See also: Rod NH, Broadbent A, Rod MH, Russo F, Arah OA, Stronks K. *Complexity in Epidemiology and Public Health. Addressing Complex Health Problems Through a Mix of Epidemiologic Methods and Data.* Epidemiology. 2023 Jul 1;34(4):505-514.

9. The Social-Ecologic Model has become standard in public health in framing conditions and forces of change. With respect to child-related issues, see especially: McLeroy KR, et al (1988) An ecological perspective on health promotion programs, Health Education Quarterly 15: 351-377.

10. See for example the comprehensive public health planning framework Theory of Change (https://www.publichealth notes.com/what-is-theory-of-change-everything-explained/); see also Hasan Mehedi (2024, May 14), Theory of Change in Designing Public Health Programs (https://www.linkedin. com/pulse/theory-change-designing-public-health-programmehedi-hasan-9mlbf/)

11. Thomas R. Frieden, 2014: Six Components Necessary for Effective Public Health Program Implementation American Journal of Public Health 104, 17-22.

12. https://www.linkedin.com/company/childrensairway-first-founda tion/about/ Both authors are members of the CAFF Advisory Board.

13. APA. Sinek, S. (2011). Start with Why. Penguin Books

14. Jiang F. Sleep and Early Brain Development. Ann Nutr Metab. 2019;75 Suppl 1:44-54. doi: 10.1159/000508055. Epub 2020 Jun 19. PMID: 32564032.

15. Diane C Lim, MD, Arezu Najafi, MD, MD, Lamia Afifi, Claudio LA Bassetti, MD, Daniel J Buysse, MD, Han, MD, Fang Birgit Högl, MD, Yohannes Adama Melaku, PhD, Charles M Morin, PhD, I Pack, MBChB, Dalva Poyares, MD, Virend K Somers, Dphil, Peter R Eastwood, PhD †, Phyllis C Zee, MD, Chandra L Jackson, PhD on behalf of the World Sleep Society Global Sleep Health Taskforce, The need to144 DR. JOHN R. FINNEGAN AND SHARON MOORE - THE ... promote sleep health in public health agendas across the globe, The LANCET, Public Health, VIEWPOINT I VOLUME 8, ISSUE 10, E820-E826, OCTOBER 2023

16. Reynolds AM, Spaeth AM, Hale L, Williamson AA, LeBourgeois MK, Wong SD, Hartstein LE, Levenson JC, Kwon M, Hart CN, Greer A, Richardson CE, Gradisar M, Clementi MA, Simon SL, Reuter-Yuill LM, Picchietti DL, Wild S, Tarokh L, Sexton-Radek K, Malow BA, Lenker KP, Calhoun SL, Johnson DA, Lewin D, Carskadon MA. Pediatric sleep: current knowledge, gaps, and opportunities for the future. Sleep. 2023

10.1093/sleep/zsad060. Jul PMID: 11;46(7):zsad060. 36881684; doi: PMCID: PMC10334737.

17. Gozal D, Tan HL, Kheirandish-Gozal L. Treatment of Obstructive Sleep Apnea in Children: Handling the Unknown with Precision. J Clin Med. 2020 Mar 24;9(3):888. doi: 10.3390/jcm9030888. PMID: 32213932; PMCID: PMC7141493.

18. Neurobehavioral Morbidity of Pediatric Mild SleepDisordered Breathing and Obstructive Sleep Apnea https://academic.oup.com/sleep/advance-article/doi/ 10.1093/sleep/zsac035/6527698

19. Isaiah A, et al. Associations between frontal lobe structure, parent-reported obstructive sleep disordered breathing and childhood behavior in the ABCD dataset. Nature Communications. DOI: 10.1038/s41467-021-22534-0 (2021).

20. Anatomy refers to the internal and external structures of the body and their physical relationships. Physiology refers to the study of the functions of those structures.

21. Faria A, Allen AH, Fox N, Ayas N, Laher I. The public health burden of obstructive sleep apnea. Sleep Sci. 2021 JulSep;14(3):257-265. doi: 10.5935/1984-0063.20200111. PMID: 35186204; PMCID: PMC8848533.

22. Bonuck K, Freeman K, Chervin RD, Xu L. Sleep-disordered breathing in a population-based cohort: behavioral outcomes at 4 and 7 years. Pediatrics. 2012;129(4): e857-e865. doi:10.1542/peds.2011-1402

23. Singaram M, Muraleedhran VR, Sivaprakasam M. Cross fertilisation of Public Health and Translational Research. J Indian Inst Sci. 2022;102(2):763-782. doi: 10.1007/s41745-022-00317-w. Epub 2022 Aug 10. PMID: 35968232; PMCID: PMC9364283.

24. Ehsan Z, Glynn EF, Hoffman MA, Ingram DG, AlShawwa B. Small sleepers, big data: leveraging big data to explore sleep-disordered breathing in infants and young children. Sleep. 2021 Feb 12;44(2): 10.1093/sleep/zsaa176. PMID: 32926133.

25. See the CAFF website at: https://www.childrensairwayfirst.org/

26. Many nations are suspicious of such global efforts wherein data are public and potentially reflect badly on a country's leadership.

27. Mehta B, et al (2020) Sleep disordered breathing (SDB) in neonates and implications for its long-term impact. Paediatric Respiratory Reviews 34 (2020) 3–8, Australia.

28. Australia. Parliament. House of Representatives. Standing Committee on Health, Aged Care and Sport & Zimmerman, Trent & Commonwealth of Austra (2019). Bedtime reading : inquiry into sleep health awareness in Australia. House of Representatives, Standing Committee on Health, Aged Care and Sport, Canberra.

29. All state panels draw from a federally recommended list for at least 29 newborn screening tests. Source: NICHD.

30. See Philip W. Cooper, DDS, (2009) Why African American Children Can Not Read, New York: iUniverse: New York describes the impact of chronic sleep apnea on rising numbers of Black children in the educa-

tional system who are labeled with ADHD and other behavioral learning disorders.

31. Tarini, Beth A., MD, MS (2007) Current Revolution in Newborn Screening: New Technology, Old Controversies. Arch Adolesc Med. 2007;161(8):767-772. doi:10.1001/archpedi.161.8.767. See also: https://www.investigatetv.com/2023/03/27/death-by-zip-code-how-statebor ders-dictate-critical-screening-newborns/

32. Fisher J, Berman R, Buse K et al, (Feb. 13, 2023) Achieving Oral Health for All through Public Health Approaches, Interprofessional, and Transdisciplinary Education, Washington DC: National Academy of Medicine.

33. Tan HL, Kaditis AG. Phenotypic variance in pediatric obstructive sleep apnea. Pediatr Pulmonol. 2021 Jun;56(6):1754-1762. doi: 10.1002/ppul.25309. Epub 2021 Feb 16. PMID: 33543838.

34. All state panels draw from a federally recommended list for at least 29 newborn screening tests. Source: NICHD.

35. APA. Bright futures pocket guide (4th ed.). (2017). American Academy of Pediatrics.

36. Buja, L. Maximilian: Medical education today: All that glitters is not gold, BMC Medical Education (2019) 19:110. https://doi.org/10.1186/s12909-019-1535-9

37. Barr H. Medicine and the making of interprofessional education. Br J Gen Pract. 2010 Apr;60(573):296-9. doi: 10.3399/bjgp10X484039. PMID: 20353679; PMCID: PMC2845496.

38. Mohammed CA, Anand R, Saleena Ummer V. Interprofessional Education (IPE): A framework for introducing teamwork and collaboration in health professions curriculum. Med J Armed Forces India. 2021 Feb;77(Suppl 1):S16-S21. doi: 10.1016/j.mjafi.2021.01.012. Epub 2021 Feb 2. PMID: 33612927; PMCID: PMC7873741.

39. Rao, Ravi, et al (2020 Jun 26), The evolving role of public health in medical education. Frontiers in Public Health, Vol 8, Article 251, doi: 10.3389/fpubh.2020.00251.

40. https://babyology.com.au/health/family-health/mums-warning-chil dren-should-not-breathe-through-their-mouths

41. https://www.thecut.com/article/halsey-revealslupus-diagnosis-new-song.html

42. Trust for America's Health: fah.org/ https://www.treports/

43. One of the first social media sites is thought to have been SixDe-grees.com appearing in 1997. It was possible to set up a personal profile, connections and networks of contacts. This was 48 months after the first "graphical" browser appeared (Mosaic).

RESOURCES

Here are five websites to help parents along at the beginning of their child's airway health journey:

www.asapathway.com
www.facefocused.com
www.wellspoken.com.au
www.airwayhealthsolutions.com
www.childrensairwayfirst.org

Books:

- "Breathe: The New Science of a Lost Art" by James Nestor
- "Breathe, Sleep, Thrive" by Dr. Shereen Lim
- "Sleep Wrecked Kids: Helping Parents Raise Happy, Healthy Kids One Sleep at a Time" by Sharon Moore
- "Why We Sleep: Unlocking the Power of Sleep and Dreams" by Matthew Walker
- "Sleep Apnea in Children: Handbook for Families" by Davide Ingram
- "ADHD 2.0" by Edward M. Hallowell & John J. Ratey, MD
- "JAWS: The Story of a Hidden Epidemic" by Sandra Kahn & Paul Ehrlich
- "Airway is Life: Waking Up to Your Family's Sleep Crisis" by Meghna Dassani MD
- "The Breathing Cure" by Patrick McKeown

ABOUT THE AUTHOR

Candy Sparks has dedicated her career to transformational leadership in both non-profit and corporate sectors. As Executive Director of A Smoke-Free Generation, she spearheaded a groundbreaking youth anti-smoking campaign endorsed by Surgeon General C. Everett Koop and supported by the Mayo Clinic, featuring influential celebrities including Prince and stars of The Cosby Show.

At Tor Dahl and Associates, she led major organizational development projects for Fortune 500 companies including AT&T, DynCorp International, and ICI, driving significant improvements in quality, efficiency, and stakeholder satisfaction. Her international impact expanded as Executive Director of the World Confederation of Productivity Science, where she organized global congresses across four continents.

Today, inspired by her daughter's struggle with a compromised airway and its systemic health effects, Candy serves as President and Co-Founder of the Children's Airway First Foundation. The foundation works to combat a silent epidemic affecting 400 million children worldwide through innovative diagnostics, interdisciplinary medical training, and public health education focused on early intervention.

A graduate of the University of Minnesota in Communications with an emphasis in Broadcast Journalism, Candy also served as a guest lecturer at the University's School of Public Health from 1986 to 2000. She and her husband Bradley

Sparks enjoy time with their five children and ten grand-children.

www.authorcandysparks.com